About

Dr Robert Erdmann, an Ameri̶c̶a̶ p̶, ... g̶... r̶... living in ̶Tunbridge Wells, has spent the past fifteen years researching amino acids as nutritional supplements and using them in his clinical work with patients. His experience using them is probably broader than anyone else in the United States.

Meirion Jones is a freelance journalist with a particular expertise in health. He is also an accomplished illustrator.

This book has been written for informational purposes only. Although the suggestions we make on how to use amino acids are based on hundreds of case histories and many years of experience in the field of amino supplementation they should not be mistaken for prescriptions. If you have doubts about taking amino acids yourself, you should seek the advice of a competent health professional.

Dedication:

To globs of amino acids in the form of future generations, to patients, and to lovers all over the world. May they enjoy the best of health.   R.E.

To Mark and Jackie.   M.J.

Acknowledgements:

Leslie Kenton, Xandria Williams, A. Kalokerinos, G. Dettman, M. Burke, Robert Cathcart III, W. Belfield, W. Shock, L. Shock, P. Emau, G. Jones, M. Erdmann, C. Shamlin, L. Rose, R. Kunin, M. Lessor, B. Belag, A. Levin, J. Patrick, I. Stone, G. Gordon.

THE AMINO REVOLUTION

Dr ROBERT ERDMANN
and
MEIRION JONES

CENTURY
LONDON MELBOURNE AUCKLAND JOHANNESBURG

First published in 1987 by Century Hutchinson Ltd
Brookmount House, 62–65 Chandos Place,
Covent Garden,London WC2N 4NW

Century Hutchinson Australia Pty Ltd
89-91 Albion Street, Surry Hills, New South Wales 2010,
Australia

Century Hutchinson New Zealand Limited
PO Box 40–086, Glenfield, Auckland 10,
New Zealand

Century Hutchinson South Africa (Pty) Ltd
PO Box 337, Bergvlei, 2012 South Africa

Typeset by Avocet Marketing Services,
Bicester, Oxon

Printed and bound in Great Britain by
The Guernsey Press Co. Ltd.,
Guernsey, Channel Islands

Reprinted 1988

British Library Cataloguing in Publication Data

Erdmann, Robert
    The amino revolution: the most exciting development in
    nutrition since the vitamin tablet.
    1. Amino acids in human nutrition
    I. Title   II. Jones, Meirion
    613.2'8   TX553.A5

ISBN 0-7126-2988-2

Table of Contents

Author's Note

My interest in nutrition, and its importance in health care, was sparked by my mother. I remember as a child hearing her say that good nutrition was vital for our wellbeing. She made the whole family take cod liver oil and would often sprinkle wheat germ on our food. Even so, at that time there was so little awareness of the dangers of refined foods that along with every other child in the neighbourhood, no sooner was I out of the house than I was stuffing my face with sweets.

Years later, following my qualification as a psychologist, I found myself drawn to the way that behaviour was influenced by food. I knew that simple things such as hunger caused loss of concentration and irritability, but what really fascinated me were tests showing how vitamin C supplements could actually raise the IQs of schoolchildren. Conversely a shortage of important nutrients was found to lower IQ, and lead to general underachievement.

It seemed obvious that, as my mother had insisted, good nutrition was essential for both physical and mental health. Yet when I tried to discuss this with my brother, a medical doctor, he told me that his entire training in nutrition had consisted of a single morning lecture. Realizing how undervalued the notion of good nutrition is in health care, but convinced of its importance, I decided to find out everything I could about the subject. I felt that the best way to learn was to devise and teach a course in 'Superhealth'. My idea was that, rather than treating peoples' illnesses, I would give healthy people the nutritional information they needed to stay healthy. My plan was to help them to avoid getting ill in the first place.

As I became more deeply involved in this idea, discovering all I could about the application of nutritional supplements, I came across the largely unexplored area of amino acid therapy. Unexplored it may have been but I quickly recognized the importance of amino acids in maintaining the vitality of mind and body. It changed the direction of my clinical practice.

Since then my understanding of the workings of the body – its breathtakingly beautiful network of metabolic pathways and its amazing resistance to illness when it is given therapeutic levels of nutrients – has grown rapidly. I believe that the benefits of taking supplements of amino acids to improve your health can hardly be overstated. All the body's tissue – every cell, muscle, hair and nail – each enzyme and each brain chemical is made from amino acids. They are central to the biochemistry of your body.

I use amino acid supplements – together with the vitamins and minerals the body needs to help metabolize them – in my nutritional counselling practice. I have come to believe that most illnesses, even viral and bacterial, result from nutritional deficiencies. The essence of my practice lies in discovering which substances are missing or in short supply, then providing them to the patient as supplements. With this philosophy – using nutritional supplementation – I have helped the victims of a wide variety of psychological complaints – from depression to anorexia and alcoholism. Equally I have found that the immune system can be supported to relieve such physical disorders as arthritis and cancer. Furthermore, by giving patients the nutrition they need to make them healthy the focus moves away from sickness to health, and what it takes to stay healthy.

This book sets out to explain my working methods, examining the theory behind nutritional counselling as well as looking at its success in practice. You'll see how different illnesses and disorders respond to different combinations of high potency amino acid supplements. I am convinced that this form of therapy, which includes vitamin and mineral co-factors, offers the best way forward for health care in the future. And I hope that after reading the book you'll agree.

Robert Erdmann, October 1986

Preface

It so often happens that our vision of search is towards the horizon, little realizing that what we are seeking lies at our own feet. We look for remedies in drugs while completely overlooking the body's need for missing nutritional links. The *cause* of malfunction is deficiency, whereas the *effect* of the malfunction may be disease. In such an instance the true method of treatment is to rectify the cause, and not to quell the effect with drugs and leave the cause untreated.

Amino acids work as body-building blocks, protectors of the cells, alleviators of pain, generators of ecstasy, the sex food for fulfilment and guardians of health. In fact the whole process of well-being depends upon them. They can shield us from the modern world's menaces of radiation and pollution, and can definitely present a way to combat the ageing process. Free amino acids can help against allergies and auto immune diseases, and can chelate the heavy metals in our body.

When I was seeking an anti-ageing programme for my clinic I turned to Dr Robert Erdmann; he is a brilliant nutritionist, and completely dedicated to his profession. He produces near miraculous results in patients and infuses a degree of wellbeing which they claim never to have enjoyed before. The answer to rejuvenation in man does not lie in the 'monkey gland' or placental extracts, but in the synergistic action of free amino acids, vitamins and minerals.

This book tells you how to increase the efficiency of your body. It is the guiding light which some will follow and some ignore, such is the nature of things. It is my pleasure to recommend this invaluable guide to wellbeing.

Mr D Basra FRCS

Foreword

by Leslie Kenton

This remarkable book speaks about the use of free-form amino acids as part of a total self-care approach to metabolic nutrition where vitamins, minerals and other natural substances are used to rectify whatever biochemical imbalances prevent someone from living at a high level of vitality and well-being. It is an approach which makes it possible not only to help an ailing body to heal itself but, even more important, to keep a well one well and to protect it from premature ageing and degenerative illness.

I first came upon some of the near-miracles which free-form amino acids could perform ten years ago when I met forward-thinking doctors in the United States using them to treat ailments as diverse as manic-depression, anxiety, poor memory, high blood pressure, sexual problems and arthritis. Ever since, I have wanted to see someone truly knowledgable about their use, produce a guide for the general public. *The Amino Revolution* is such a guide – and responsibly so for it never advocates the use of these potent building blocks of nature without full nutritional support from the co-factor vitamins and minerals necessary to make efficient and safe use of them as part of a total nutritional programme.

To stay alive and healthy the body continuously uses energy. This energy, which has its ultimate origins in the sun, is made available to us thanks to the special biochemical transformations which we as living creatures are able to perform. In a young and healthy body these transformations are carried out in miraculously ordered ways thanks to a supply of raw materials – vitamins, minerals, amino-acids, essential fatty acids and other metabolites – being available in abundance. Interwoven, interacting and interdependent in highly elaborate ways, these biochemical transformations make the world's most advanced computer look like a child's toy. Each takes place in a series of chemical steps. These chemical chains of events which begin with a single molecule and proceed by changing one thing into another until your body has made the specific substance it needs for a particular purpose are known as metabolic pathways – the means by which all life processes are carried out. And the healthy human body is a biological masterpiece. It has superbly balanced mechanisms which rise to the occasion when you are sick and keep you ticking over when you are well. Erdmann and Jones understand well that high level health depends entirely upon maintaining such a dynamic biochemical balance. When something goes wrong with the balance – either as a result of stress or poor diet or microbial invasion – then illness ensues. Just what kind of illness and just how serious depends upon your inherited weaknesses and on the strength of your immune system.

The Erdmann-Jones metabolic approach to nutrition attempts to supply your body with what it needs to maintain its own health or to heal itself from within. This it does by making sure that as many as possible of the body's highly complex metabolic pathways have the specific nutrients they require in optimal amounts to function smoothly and efficiently.

Their book is based on an extremely simple yet profound nuts and bolts hypothesis which goes something like this: our bodies are quite literally constructed out of vitamins, minerals, amino acids, fatty acids, and other metabolites derived from them, working together according to a living molecular logic. Because we are alive, that life provides us with the consciousness to utilize these nuts and bolts via this elaborate network of superbly engineered and interlocking metabolic pathways. So, if we can discover exactly which nuts and bolts in the form of vitamins and minerals, amino acids and essential fatty acids are needed in extraordinary amounts, or are simply in short supply in your body and then to be able to top them up, all will be well.

Erdmann himself is an extraordinary combination of in-depth knowledge and highly developed intuition and inventiveness. His co-author Meirion Jones is a young man of exceptional intelligence with the ability to put into simple and often highly amusing language even the most complex information. Together, I believe they have written a book which will be of enormous help to anyone, well or unwell, who has asked the question 'How can I look and feel better than I do right now?'

Introduction

The introduction of amino acids in the form of powders, pill or capsules is the most exciting advance in health and nutrition for twenty-five years. This book shows you why. In the following pages you'll see how, they can be used to improve both mental and physical vitality. As dieting supplements they ease pain, soothe anxiety, combat viruses and even heighten sexual performance.

Aminos and the body

Amino acids aren't a new medical discovery. In fact in their natural state, as the building blocks of protein, they form the basis of life itself. They are the essential raw materials in the growth and reproduction of every cell of your body. Selected aminos are present in your enzymes and immune system. Every bone, organ and muscle and almost all hormones are made from combinations of aminos often with the help of vitamins and minerals.

Until recently most doctors believed that taking supplements of pure – or 'free form' as they are called – amino acids as a means of improving health was unnecessary. After all, they reasoned, as most diets are so abundant in protein it's likely that we can get all the amino acids we need simply from the food we eat. Admittedly in a perfect world this would be true. Unfortunately in our imperfect one countless factors work to prevent our bodies from receiving a full and balanced supply of these all-important substances: in our rivers and in the air, the pollution the hormones fed to cattle, the intensive use of fertilisers in agriculture and even habits such as smoking and drinking can all prevent our bodies from making full use of what we eat.

Worse still is the amount of nutrition which is lost from our food through processing before we actually get to eat it. This danger is illustrated by a famous experiment into the effects of food processing conducted by Professor Francis Pottenger. Taking two groups of kittens he fed one group on fresh meat, the other on an exclusive diet of tinned (processed) cat food. In time the kittens in both groups grew to maturity and produced litters of their own. With each succeeding generation the cats fed on fresh food flourished – their fur was glossy and sleek, their behaviour lively and alert. The cats in the tinned food group, on the other hand, suffered a gradual physical and mental deterioration – growth was stunted, they became increasingly psychotic and unsociable and were eventually unable to reproduce.

Of course our diets are much more varied than those used in this controlled experiment – we eat a diversity of meat, dairy products and vegetables. Nevertheless it suggests that no matter how nutritious or tasty our food seems we may still not be receiving everything we need for a healthy, balanced lifestyle. And if in doubt you only have to look for proof at the rise in the incidences of cancer, heart disease, nervous breakdowns and anxiety neuroses. This is where free-form amino acid supplements come in. By providing the body with optimal nutrition, amino acids help to replace what is lost and in doing so promote wellbeing and vitality.

Pathways and stop-signs

As you read through the book you'll realize that an important key to using amino acids is possessing a clear understanding of what health really means. By the standards of conventional medicine it is defined as the absence of disease – when there are no identifiable symptoms of illness the patient is said to be well. By the same token when an illness does occur it is often treated as an isolated phenomenon which has arisen independent of the rest of the body. In these cases drugs are prescribed to suppress the symptoms often without any thought of the deeper and longer-term consequences.

Using amino acids on the other hand means adopting a radically different attitude. It means considering the inner workings of your body, where the reactions of each individual chemical cause reactions elsewhere. These reactions are called metabolic pathways and you will be reading about them a lot in this book. Metabolic pathways are the body's biochemical assembly lines which take the raw materials from your food and manufacture finished products to help the body to live. These finished products include everything from enzymes for digestion and brain chemicals which let us think, to organs, bones and teeth. Making certain that the metabolic pathways work at peak performance – meeting your body's precise molecular demands – means ensuring that your body has all the raw materials it needs: vitamins, minerals fatty acids and, most important of all, amino acids. Using amino acids to treat symptoms of an illness therefore, is really only a green light signalling the start of a journey that leads deep into the miraculous world of the metabolic pathways. In this book we'll be taking many such journeys.

The heart of the matter

So what can amino acids offer that conventional medicine can't? Can they claim to be on the threshold of an AIDS vaccine breakthrough? Have they pioneered the use of brain scans? No in both cases. Instead what the use of amino acids is showing is something that in its own way is just as valuable. It is making people aware of their bodies as the supremely harmonious organisms that they are. It is showing how every disorder, each faltering loss of vitality and wellbeing, is the result of metabolic imbalances rather than a single specific cause. It is showing how the illnesses these imbalances cause can be cured with nutritional supplementation. In other words, with extra supplements of the raw materials found in the food we eat every day of our lives – that is, amino acids, together with certain vitamins and minerals – we can enhance our health and vitality as never before.

In 'The Amino Revolution' you'll be seeing what this means in practice. By examining the metabolic imbalances behind a variety of health problems we'll find out which aminos are involved. Then, by suggesting specific combinations of individual free form aminos you'll see how to restore balance to the affected pathway. In this way you can strengthen your immune system against infection and disease, restore emotional and mental balance, overcome the bad habits of a lifetime (such as smoking) and generally create enormous vitality – enough to meet all the immense demands of the twentieth century.

If you are used to thinking of improving your health by taking a single pill – such as vitamin C for a cold, or worse, a drug which only suppresses the cold's symptoms – this new amino-based approach could radically alter your attitude and expectations. Used wisely amino acids supplements are miracles of nature. They are safe, simple and unequalled among natural substances for their health-enhancing potential. The title of this book is no exaggeration. Thanks to amino acids we are poised at the edge of a revolution in health.

PART ONE

MEET THE FREE AMINOS

Chapter 1

The Aminos in Person

The twenty-four hour endurance race at the Spa circuit in Belgium is second only to Le Mans for the demands it makes on competitors. Although a team of three drivers takes turns at manning each car, the race is a gruelling test of will and strength. This was especially true during the July 1986 race for one driver, Allan Moffat. With a team-mate withdrawing half-way through the race from heat exhaustion, Moffat was forced to drive two shifts in a row. The stifling heat, the cabin reverberating with engine noise, the almost superhuman level of concentration and the continuous gear changes demanded more from him than anyone had a right to expect. Yet, thanks in large part to Allan's driving, his team received many of the after-race trophies, including the prestigious Kings' Cup.

The most remarkable thing about this drive is that, only a matter of days before, Allan had been ill, the victim of a debilitating, six-week-long virus infection. During this period he had endured such a bad headache that at times he thought his eyes 'would force their way of of my head'. On top of this he was constantly tired and felt his strength fading by the day. Antibiotics had done nothing but make him sleepy, and as the day of the race approached he feared that he would have to drop out for the good of the team.

Then, with only a few days to go, Allan came for nutritional counselling. Explaining his problem, he asked if anything could be done at such short notice to prepare him physically for the race. He was immediately put on a high potency nutritional formula which included vitamins and minerals. The single most important part of this blend, though, was a selection of certain amino acid supplements. These aminos were specially chosen to boost his energy levels, giving him the vitality both to withstand the stresses of the race and to stave off the effects of the virus. They worked so well that, in addition to covering for his co-driver, he was the only member of his team with enough strength left to collect their trophies. As his wife said later, 'I've never seen him look so good after a race in all the years I've known him.'

Allan's case isn't an isolated one. More and more people are finding that supplementing their diets with amino acids is one of the most effective and thorough ways of ensuring their health and vitality. Free-form amino acids (that is, amino acids which have been separated in the laboratory from their parent protein molecules) are being hailed as one of the greatest advances in medical care this century. The aim of this book is to explain why this claim is anything but extravagant.

In later chapters – quoting up-to-the minute research and the case histories of many people whose physical and mental illnesses amino acids have relieved – we'll show you how to use these remarkable substances. Whether you suffer from mood disorders such as depression and anxiety, illnesses such as peptic ulcers, virus infections or heart problems, whether you have difficulty slimming, find it impossible to stop smoking or drinking, or simply have a sieve-like memory, amino acids can help you.

But before all this let's find out exactly what amino acids are. How do they work in the body? Why is amino acid supplementation so effective? As amino acids are involved in almost every living function of your body, answering these questions means having to explore the way your skin and bones are formed, how organs function and what enables you to grow, regenerate and resist disease. It means taking a journey deep into the miraculous living processes of your body.

The Metabolic Republic

Your body is an incredibly complex organism. Imagine it for a moment as a massive self-contained city. It really isn't such a fanciful comparison. Your cells, after all, are a teeming population of many races and occupations. The arteries are a network of main roads used constantly by high-speed couriers, taxis, heavy goods vehicles and dustcarts. Like any city, there are different means of communicating. There are factories, supermarkets, power stations and beautifully designed architectural wonders; it can even boast its own civil defence militia. Although these examples are actually enzymes, hormones, the nervous system, the liver and antibodies, they serve the same purpose in your body as their equivalents in a city. There is, however, one flaw in this comparison; cities are randomly gathered groupings of people and institutions each working for their own separate interests. Everything in your body, on the other hand, exists and works solely for one purpose – to keep you alive and healthy. This means a constant process of renewal, of clearing away debris and building anew, of fighting disease and repairing damage. And this process can only take place if the body receives sufficient nutrition.

The Nutrients of Life

Your food comes in three basic forms: carbohydrates, fats and proteins. The first two are very simply structured. Carbohydrate, for example, exists only as a few variations of glucose and fructose. It contributes only slightly to your wellbeing and most of what you need can be made in the body itself. Fats are almost as simple. They take the form of lecithin or cholesterol; or as three fat molecules combined, which are called triglycerides. The third, protein, is very different.

The word 'protein' is Greek and means 'first things'. Three-quarters of all the solid matter in your body is protein. While there are only three or four forms each of fat and carbohydrate in the human body, there are at least fifty thousand recognised forms of protein. This enormous number of differing protein structures gives your body the range and versatility which it needs to live. Unlike fat or carbohydrate, protein is absolutely essential for life – to build all the different parts of its 'city'. All enzymes and most hormones, every cell and muscle and every piece of tissue from blood vessel to eyeball are made of protein. Without it we would have no teeth and bones, no nervous system, no life.

To live and grow our bodies need this huge number of different proteins. Moreover, each of these proteins must be custom-built to specifications which are peculiar to your body and to no one else's. Simply reusing the protein you eat would never meet these specifications. To give you an idea why, imagine an architect dismantling Stonehenge in order to build an ornate mansion from the stone. Obviously it would be impossible to use the massive granite slabs as they are. So before his builders can go to work the slabs have to be broken apart and chiselled into various shapes to form keystones, sills and fluting. Only when this process is finished can the segments of rock be reconstructed to make the house. In the same way, the protein you eat is broken up into smaller constituents and then remade in a different form to meet your body's exact needs. These tiny constituent parts, the building blocks of your body, are amino acids.

In breaking down and then reconstructing the protein you eat your body can produce over fifty thousand different protein structures. Yet there are only twenty-two constituent amino acids. How can they produce so many variations? The answer lies in the

5

one crucial difference between the molecules of amino acids and those of fats and carbohydrates. While all three contain atoms of carbon, hydrogen and oxygen, amino acids contain nitrogen as well. An amino acid is basically a 'Y' shape. One branch of the 'Y' contains the amino group; the other contains the acid. The tail, known as the 'R' group, contains the nitrogen, sometimes with sulphur, and it is this tail which gives protein its enormous versatility.

When your body needs a particular protein, the amino acids needed to make it are linked together in a chain. The amino branch of one molecule joins with the acid branch of the next and the link is bonded by enzymes called peptides. Amino-acid chains are therefore sometimes called polypeptides rather than proteins. No matter how many amino acids join together, there are always branches free to make further bonds. Protein molecules have been found which contain chains of as many as five hundred amino acids – many, of course, are the same type but bonded in specific sequences. Each time another amino acid is added, the chain becomes a new and separate protein with different properties and different functions in the body. This is what makes one polypeptide chain a digestive enzyme and another, with possibly only a slightly different sequence of amino acids, a molecule of muscle fibre tissue.

The ability to create either highly active chemicals or hard, fibrous structures shows the versatility of amino-based proteins. But for all their variety, they are still only chains – minute molecular strands. How do these fragile chains form the complex and robust structures of your body? Picture a beautifully trimmed hedge, surrounding a lawn on three sides. It is so well tended that it looks like one continuous plant – almost a solid wall. In fact, we know it is made up of many smaller plants whose branches have become closely intertwined. The same holds true for protein molecules. By cross-linking and intertwining with other molecule chains of the same protein, they form multi-layered latticeworks. Then, folding back on themselves, forming loops and super-imposing themselves on other latticeworks, they gradually build up into the highly complicated and specialized three-dimensional structures that make up everything in your body, from teeth to nerve fibres. Carbohydrates and fats can't do this, which is why protein – the product of an almost limitless number of amino acid combinations – is so vital. Without it life would simply not be.

The spiral path

Now let's look at these three-dimensional protein formations a little more closely. They are divided into two basic groups – fibrous protein and globular protein. As its name suggests, fibrous protein creates essentially solid, straight tissue such as muscle. The simplest form of this protein is called fibroin. It is made from straight amino acid chains and has very little three-dimensional structuring. Silk is made from fibroin and it's this simple form that gives it its almost watery flimsiness. Fibroin was one of the two proteins used in the ground-breaking experiments into protein structure by Professor W. Astbury at Leeds University; the other protein he used was keratin, the main constituent of fingernails and toenails. As nails are so much stronger and more robust than silk, Astbury assumed that keratin was the more complex of the two proteins. However, after soaking keratin in water, he found that it could be stretched to twice its original length. When he compared X-rays of the stretched keratin with those of fibroin he found that their molecular structures were almost identical – in both cases they were straight and two-dimensional. So what was it that made fibroin flimsy and keratin hard?

The question was answered by the Nobel-prize-winning biochemist, Linus Pauling. He discovered that in its natural form keratin was actually helix-shaped – it resembled a spiral staircase. It's now known that all fibrous proteins, except for fibroin, display this helix shape. Separate helixes can join together like spliced rope to give the molecule extra strength. And the more complex the protein becomes, the more strands are woven together. This leads to the creation of collagen for skin tissue, elastin for tendons and actin and myosin for muscles. Organs and glands, blood vessels and nerve endings all depend on these helix shapes. Even bones are made from a latticework of amino-based fibrous protein, with calcium phosphate filling in the holes.

The other basic form of protein, globular protein, is somewhat different. Unlike the fibrous protein structures that are laid down wherever needed in compact strips of interwoven chains, globular molecules are often composed of single chains which fold and curl back on themselves like a ball of wool. These proteins are normally found within the cells and serve very different functions from their fibrous counterparts.

Remember, fibrous protein creates heavy, substantial structures. They perform their mechanical tasks according to given stimuli. When a muscle flexes, for example, or a blood vessel dilates, they are obeying orders from the brain. It is the globular proteins, as enzymes and hormones, which relay these orders. Globular proteins create soluble, highly reactive chemicals.

Enzymes are usually made with the help of vitamins and minerals. For our bodies to work – for muscles to contract, capillaries to dilate, digestion to occur and orders to be carried from the brain to the rest of the body – enzymes cause thousands of chemical reactions to take place every second. If a scientist were to try to copy a single one of these reactions in his laboratory, he would need the intense heat of a bunsen burner, high pressure and a potent acid or alkali – all acting as catalysts – together with an amazingly sensitive measuring device to judge the precise amount of chemicals to be used. Then the entire process – measuring the individual chemicals, applying the catalyst and reaching the finished product – would have to be accomplished in the split second it takes an enzyme to do the same thing in our bodies. Enzymes pick up two or more of the chemicals which the body needs to react, bringing them together to create a new substance. They are made of three-dimensional amino acid bundles with slots, rather like plug sockets, into which one set of reacting chemicals fits.

Now let's imagine that our scientist wants to take his experiments a step further. Instead of copying a single reaction, he decides to stimulate every one of the thousands of reactions that occur in our bodies continuously. To do so he will have to construct a fabulous jungle of furnaces and storage tanks feeding a spaghetti junction of interconnecting pipes. Every time two of these pipes meet, the chemicals inside – an enzyme in one, perhaps, and an amino acid in the other – react to produce a new substance. Sometimes newly created substances are involved in further reactions which produce other substances.

Instead of an imaginary Heath Robinson contraption of pipes, the complex biochemical transformations that occur in your body are known as metabolic pathways. You will be hearing a lot about them in the following pages. For while amino acids are the raw materials, metabolic pathways are the assembly lines which manufacture finished products. Using reacting enzymes, these pathways forge the aminos into substances that will be used to structure bones and teeth, the brain chemicals that let us think and even other enzymes – both for digestion and metabolic pathways. Ensuring that these pathways work at peak performance – that they meet the body's precise demands – means giving your body all the amino acids it needs.

Of course, ensuring that all these reactions take place at all is a stupendous task. The brain has to coordinate the continuous chemical production, bringing together the right chemicals with enzymes which have themselves been made from other reactions. It also has to cope with the unexpected. To do so the body relies on biochemical messengers to activate the enzymes. These are called hormones and most are also made from globular proteins. Hormones order the body to grow, trigger puberty, make you happy or excited or sad. They even tell you when you're hungry.

Blueprints of Metabolism

Let's now imagine a group of newly-digested aminos ready to be used somewhere in the body. What mechanism is going to oversee their construction as a specific protein, assembling them in the correct sequence of numbers? Every cell manufactures several thousand new proteins a minute. Even a minor change in the way that the aminos are linked could result in illness or mutation. So there must be a process which ensures correct bonding. Although the job of enzymes is to link different aminos, and of hormones to order any process to begin, they could never meet the huge demands themselves. Instead there are two substances which exist solely for this purpose – dioxy-ribonucleic acid (DNA) and ribonucleic acid (RNA). These two nucleic acids, widely distributed in human tissue, play a major role in heredity as well as in protein synthesis. DNA can be looked upon as the blueprint of the entire body. It is a double-helix which contains every piece of information on the way the body is built, encoded into its strands like the holes of a piano roll. One part of this 'roll' might tell you which aminos and enzymes are needed for a piece of skin tissue, another for the manufacture of a white blood cell. This is called the genetic code. And as the nucleus of each cell contains DNA every bit of information can be found in every cell.

While DNA contains all the information of body structure, RNA acts like a metabolic index. If the body needs, say, some muscle fibre, the RNA discovers the part of the DNA masterplan which contains the information needed for the relevant piece of protein synthesis. The RNA then attaches itself to this section. Think of a sheet of plastic being vacuum-moulded and you get an idea of the replication process that occurs next. The RNA assumes the shape of this part of the DNA, becoming in fact an exact copy. This copy is known as a ribosome. Detaching itself from the DNA, it acts as a template for protein synthesis, attracting and binding the amino acids in the correct number and sequence according to the code it has copied from the DNA. The completed molecule can then be added wherever it is needed.

When Things Go Wrong

Protein synthesis takes place continuously almost everywhere in the body. It seems to be such a precise operation – the different substances all reacting together in harmony – that it might easily lull you into thinking that nothing could possibly go awry. But you'd be wrong. The very fact that your body is such a delicate and exact mechanism leaves it vulnerable to a vast number of factors. These only need affect you in seemingly minor ways to disrupt the metabolic harmony, leaving you prone to illness and disorder.

Imagine for a moment that you have bad teeth. Perhaps your dentures don't fit or you suffer from an aching molar. For whatever reason you are forced to swallow your food without chewing it properly. Normally chewing tears your food apart enabling the digestive substances to attack a large surface area. The more thoroughly you chew the greater the amount of nutrients your body will absorb. On the other hand inadequate chewing leaves a smaller surface area of the food available for the acids and enzymes to work on and when it reaches the gut less of it is digested. Because of this fewer amino acids are absorbed into the body to carry out the vital protein synthesis. As one of the important roles of protein synthesis is to manufacture digestive enzymes, it means there will inevitably be fewer enzymes to digest the food. With this enzyme depletion worsening the problems created by inadequate chewing, fewer amino acids will be released from the food, further depleting the enzyme supply.

Of course, digestive enzymes won't be the only thing to suffer. As we've seen, different combinations of amino acids are needed to perform different functions in the body. As they become depleted these functions will be carried out inadequately. Sooner or later hormone production will drop: there will be less insulin to regulate your blood sugar levels, less adrenalin to help you cope with stress, less thyroxin to carry out body metabolism and less thymosin to stimulate your immune system. As supplies of the aminos which form fibrous proteins are reduced, your nails will get softer and start to split, your skin will lose its pliability and muscle tone will fade. Fats which depend on proteins to be mobilized will start to build up in the blood vessels, leading to higher blood pressure. You will get tired easily, find everyday situations stressful and suffer from periods of anxiety and depression. You will become much more susceptible to disease. You will age prematurely. At best, the quality of your life will be much lower than it should. At worst, you will die.

This picture – suggesting that you can suffer from mental and

10

physical illness simply from one loose molar – might seem a bit extreme. It is, but not by much. It shows how dependent the body is on a balanced supply of amino acids, and how easily an imbalance can be caused, affecting areas of the body that would seem to have no connection at all with your loose filling or oversized denture. And there are many factors besides bad teeth that will lead to this digestive imbalance. You could make a long list of factors that included emotional stress, junk food, inadequate exercise, viruses, pollution, injury, drug-taking (marijuana plays havoc with the secretion of stomach acid) and genetic disorders which affect protein synthesis. They will all decrease the output of digestive chemicals, which will in turn cause a snowball effect as other, unrelated disorders take hold throughout the body. If you're not nutritionally prepared to face them they can set in motion a destructive chain which will quickly spiral out of control.

This is where amino acid supplements come in. We've seen how important these building blocks of protein are to the body. We'll look at which foods contain which aminos in chapter 3. However, rather than having to depend simply on the protein you get from the food you eat to protect you from illness, you can now supplement your diet with amino supplements choosing from powders, capsules or tablets. They contain nothing but pure individual amino acids. By learning how disorders affect the different metabolic pathways of your body, we can relieve the disorder by using free-form amino acids to replenish and support the pathways. Thanks to this free-form approach we need never suffer a shortage of any vital substance. If, for example, you wanted to cure the digestive trouble started by your bad tooth, you could take a supplement containing a blend of those particular amino acids which your body uses to make its digestive enzymes. In its free-form state this blend is absorbed straight into the body, regardless of digestive difficulties. Here the pancreas can use it to manufacture all the enzymes needed to digest your food properly.

With the relevant blends of aminos this method is equally effective for mood disorders, skin complaints, virus infections, heart disease, premature ageing and cravings for alcohol and cigarettes. All these problems, after all, result from metabolic pathways having been disrupted by nutritional deficiencies. The key to relieving these disorders is to discover which amino deficiencies are responsible for which disorder. Then, by adding supplements of those aminos to our diets – together with the important vitamin and mineral co-factors (which are often needed by the body to help the conversion process of the metabolic pathways) – we can cure it. This is the theory that lies at the heart of free-form amino acid therapy.

11

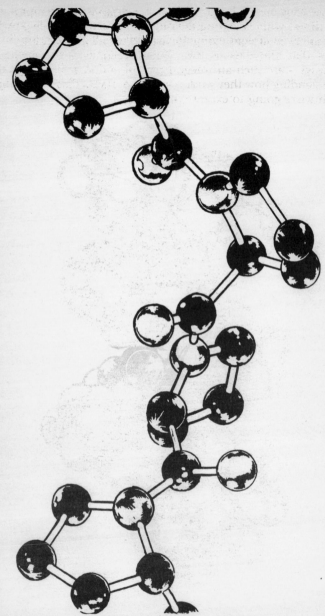

The conformation of a single strand of a collagen helix made from amino acids.

Amino acids aren't drugs. They won't suppress the symptoms of your illness while avoiding the causes. These remarkable powders work solely by strengthening the natural metabolic reactions in our bodies that allow us to live. These reactions – the metabolic pathways – are such an integral part of amino acid therapy that understanding how they work is very important. This is the subject which we're going to explore in chapter 2.

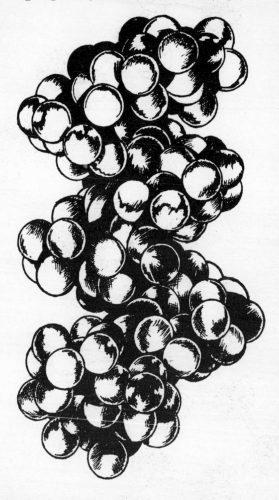

In this drawing three single strands have wound around each other, in effect 'splicing' to form a helical collagen cable.

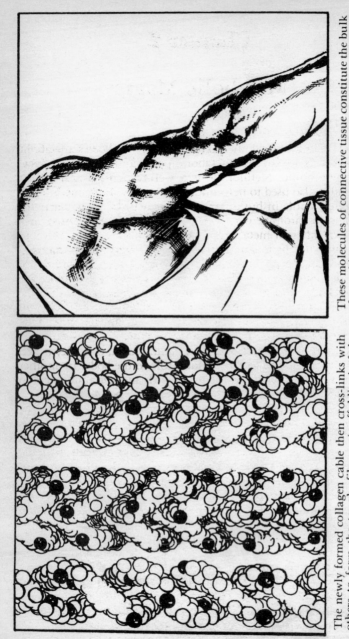

These molecules of connective tissue constitute the bulk of our skin, muscles, organs and hair as well as a large part of the structure of our bones.

The newly formed collagen cable then cross-links with others to form the tough, fibrous 'scaffolding' of the body's connective tissue.

Chapter 2

Metabolic Magic

In order to understand the complexity of the body's metabolic pathways let's follow the metabolic pathway of an amino acid called methionine. Methionine is a well-recognized anti-fatigue agent and is also used to help improve memory. First, methionine plays a major role in building protein structures, particularly the skin. The methionine which isn't used here is then used in a number of different metabolic pathways. In one it reacts with an enzyme activated by magnesium and water – three 'paths' meeting at once – to produce a substance called s-adenosyl methionine (for further details see p. 27). This is known as 'activated' methionine and the body uses it to assist many reactions. After this the methionine may be converted into one of several different substances depending on the body's needs at the time. One substance, for example, is called homocysteine. This in turn reacts with vitamin B6 to produce another amino acid, cysteine, which has a different, but no less important, role in the body. In another pathway s-adenosyl methionine reacts with another amino acid to produce the 'fight or flight' chemical adrenalin.

By causing substances to react and thereby create new ones, the metabolic pathways of your body also help to clear it of certain toxic chemicals. The best example of this is a pathway called the urea cycle. In this several different amino acids are able to create, with the appropriate vitamins and minerals, an amino called glutamic acid. This reacts in turn with the highly poisonous metabolic waste-product, ammonia, to produce glutamine – a brain fuel and natural stimulant – and urea, which can then be safely excreted (see p. 38).

These metabolic pathways can almost be thought of as maps. They show the direction that amino acids, vitamins and minerals take, telling us which substances are needed for which transformations. And because all the products of metabolic pathways are vital to the body, illness is caused when these transformations are prevented from occurring. To see more clearly how this happens let's look at another metabolic pathway. This time it starts from one of the most important amino acids of all: tryptophan.

Before entering the pathway, a certain amount of tryptophan, in common with methionine and most aminos, is used as it is for the creation of structural protein. Some is also sent to the bone marrow for the antibody-building response of your immune system. When these needs are satisfied tryptophan is transformed by a two-stage metabolic pathway into a hormone called 5-hydroxytryptamine – which we'll call by its simpler name, serotonin. This is an inhibitory neurotransmitter – a brain chemical which is responsible for sending us to sleep at night, relaxing us during the day, preventing us from overreacting to stress and guarding against inordinate rises in blood pressure. Serotonin is even involved in the reddening, swelling and flushing of our immune response when we catch cold or have an allergy. In order to convert to serotonin, tryptophan – it's precursor – needs to react with the vitamins B6 and C. But there are many factors in life, including cigarette smoke and alcohol, which work to destroy these co-factors. When this happens the metabolic pathway becomes blocked and there simply isn't enough serotonin produced to meet our needs. The results are insomnia and increasing tension and anxiety. In the longer term it might lead to chronic depression and a possible rise in blood pressure.

Inadequate tryptophan metabolism is indicated by a rise in the levels of a substance called xanthurenic acid in the urine. From this, together with the symptoms we've mentioned, nutritionists are able to deduce that the victim is suffering from a deficiency of vitamins B6 and C – the main converting substances – and, of course, serotonin. The obvious remedy is to take a free-form supplement of tryptophan together with its vitamin co-factors.

But wait. Tryptophan has other metabolic pathways, too. One is a more complex, multi-stage process resulting in the production of nicotinamide-adenine dinucleotide (NAD), a form of vitamin B3. This pathway is really a metabolic fail-safe mechanism. B3 is such an important substance in the body that if its normal sources are blocked the body will use tryptophan to create it instead. In doing so, tryptophan will be diverted away from its usual serotonin-producing pathway.

Now we see that in addition to the insomnia, anxiety and other symptoms resulting from a possible lack of tryptophan, and vitamins B6 and C, even supplying these substances in abundance may not relieve the problems. They might be caused as an indirect result of B3 deficiency. Therefore, to cover all the alternatives and ensure that each pathway is as well supplied as possible you would add a supplement of vitamin B3 to the others.

Just as tryptophan supplements will help to relieve the symptoms caused by serotonin deficiency, so understanding the metabolic pathways helps us to choose other amino acids for the different ailments we suffer from. And because vitamins and minerals are usually important in helping these stage-by-stage transformations to occur they should always be taken with the aminos.

Putting to the test

From the start we've tried to stress how complex and sensitive to change your body is. Variations from an optimal, fully nutritious diet – serving all your metabolic needs – occur very easily. Exclusively vegetarian diets, for example, are often deficient in tryptophan. As well as these functions of tryptophan which we've already looked at – producing serotonin and vitamin B3 – another pathway which suffers from this deficiency is one which produces a substance called piccolinic acid. This is a molecule the body uses to transport zinc across the gut wall. So a tryptophan deficiency will lead to less circulating zinc. This could cause an unhealthy rise in the metals which compete with it for absorption: copper and iron. This is only one of several imbalances resulting from insufficient tryptophan. And tryptophan is only one of many amino acids. With such a complex metabolic interrelationship illness can occur frighteningly easily. To try and anticipate the disorders that amino deficiencies cause, some enlightened doctors and nutritionists are now introducing highly accurate methods of nutritional testing. And by using the results from these tests a patient can start actively to manipulate his metabolism, anticipating an illness before it occurs and taking the relevant supplement of aminos to avoid it.

Probably the best test of this kind uses what is called a 'Quantitive Urinary Amino Acid Screening'. For this a patient is required to collect samples of every urination during a twenty-four-hour period. As a natural process of filtering by the kidneys, a certain amount of all the nutrients in your body are spilled into the urine – amino acids being no exception. Collecting samples for twenty-four hours takes into account the body's full metabolic cycle. From this twenty-four-hour collection the nutritionist or doctor will find traces of most amino acids. By comparing the amounts contained in these traces with the expected average, the nutritionist can discover the presence of any imbalances and blockages in the metabolic pathways and of any shortages of amino acids, vitamins and minerals. It acts very much as a metabolic X-ray, identifying the problem, pinpointing the cause and suggesting a remedy.

The results of this urinary screening are obtained by using

complex technology – a combination of chemical, electrical and mechanical engineering. First the urine is centifruged to separate unwanted protein constituents. The main instrument in the test is called a High Pressure Liquid Chromantography (HPLC) unit. Very simply, it is a measured column filled with beads of resin ions into which is injected a small but precise amount of the centrifruged urine sample. The urine is then subjected to high pressure (exceeding 1000 pounds a square inch) and a strong acid environment. During the three and a half hours which the sample is kept in the column the acidity is gradually reduced. At the same time the aminos traverse the sample and start to escape from the column through a special filtering device. As the pressure mounts (the electrically charged resin and the acid in the column affect every amino differently) each amino travels through the column at a different, prejudged rate, emerging in that period at a time peculiar to itself and to no other. In this way scientists know how long it will take, say, our friend tryptophan to emerge. As it comes out it is mixed with a dyeing chemical. The density of the dye colour that results will depend on the levels of the amino acid which were contained in the urine. An electronic eye measures the density of each dyed amino and information is fed into a computer. This then prints out a chart showing the levels of each amino present in the urine.

Let's imagine the urine sample was found to contain low levels of tryptophan. Knowing how tryptophan affects the body (especially in its serotonin-producing pathway), you could predict possible symptoms such as depression, anxiety, hypertension and insomnia – as well as the consequences of zinc deficiency. Then, instead of waiting for them to happen, you could supplement your diet with free-form tryptophan together with the important co-factors of vitamins B3, B6, C and zinc.

The insights that these tests give into the way that metabolic pathways are blocked and retarded are proving immensely beneficial in helping people to avoid a vast array of nutritionally-related problems. They also give the most accurate possible diagnosis of the problem (rather than simply examining the symptom, which is the common practice) when an illness does occur. As yet these tests are relatively expensive, but the price is dropping as more laboratories start to offer them to people.

Despite their expense and annoying impracticality, many patients over the years both in Britain and the United States have used these tests. The results have not only proved to be an excellent way of relieving health problems but have also enabled experts to extend their research and broaden their expertise in the use of amino

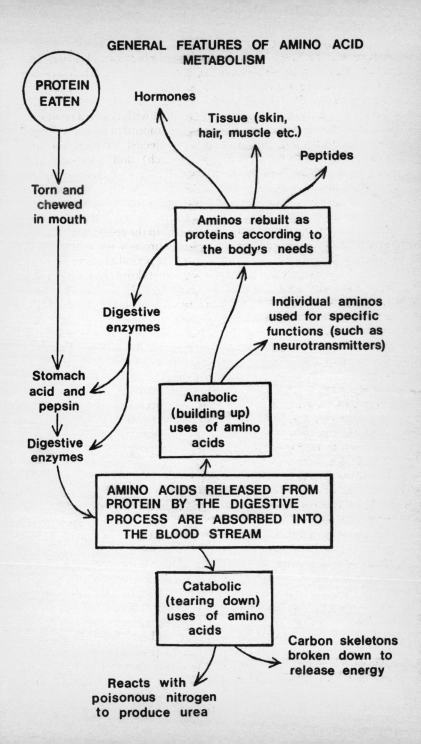

GENERAL FEATURES OF AMINO ACID METABOLISM

PROTEIN EATEN

Hormones

Tissue (skin, hair, muscle etc.)

Peptides

Torn and chewed in mouth

Aminos rebuilt as proteins according to the body's needs

Digestive enzymes

Individual aminos used for specific functions (such as neurotransmitters)

Stomach acid and pepsin

Anabolic (building up) uses of amino acids

Digestive enzymes

AMINO ACIDS RELEASED FROM PROTEIN BY THE DIGESTIVE PROCESS ARE ABSORBED INTO THE BLOOD STREAM

Catabolic (tearing down) uses of amino acids

Carbon skeletons broken down to release energy

Reacts with poisonous nitrogen to produce urea

TRYPTOPHAN IN THE BODY

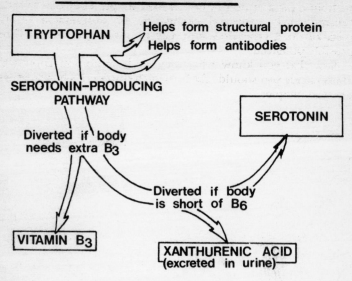

TRYPTOPHAN

Helps form structural protein
Helps form antibodies

SEROTONIN–PRODUCING
PATHWAY

SEROTONIN

Diverted if body
needs extra B₃

Diverted if body
is short of B₆

VITAMIN B₃

XANTHURENIC ACID
(excreted in urine)

acids as dietary supplements. More is now known about the individual uses of free-form amino acids than ever before and this knowledge is rapidly being passed on to the public. Tryptophan, for example, is already widely used for its power as a relaxant. Another DL-phenylalanine, is used to relieve pain and lift the depression and tension of pre-menstrual syndrome and the mood problems of menopause. These and many other amino acids are playing an ever-increasing role in health today.

Although the only way to get a really precise picture of the needs of your metabolism is through professional counselling with tests such as HPLC, you can also use amino acids yourself to develop a programme which suits you. Some people have expressed doubts about such a free rein. This is because of the idea, so firmly embedded in our society, that the only way to relieve illness is by using drugs. They find it difficult to believe that they can, if they choose, solve many of their problems themselves simply with the basic constituents of the food they eat every day of their lives – amino acids. A good example of this is the woman who reluctantly came for nutritional counselling to cure her frigidity. When a certain amino acid was recommended she said: 'I don't know what I dislike more, this inability to orgasm or having to take drugs to get over it.' She simply misunderstood what amino acids are. They're not drugs and they're non-toxic, which is why you can buy them without a prescription in health food shops. They don't work by causing some unnatural change in, or suppression of, your metabolism. All they do is simply help your body to live to its fullest possible potential.

Now that you know what they are how do you know which amino acids you should take for which disorder? The answer is in the next chapter.

Chapter 3

Get to Know the Free Aminos

The way that nutritional deficiencies affect the body can be compared with one of those spectacular attempts on the domino-falling record. To mount their attempt the organizers arrange the dominoes in a pattern, with many rows radiating out from the starting point. When the first domino is pushed over it causes several rows to topple at once, until dominoes are falling simultaneously all around the room. The same holds true of the body's metabolic pathways. A single minor deficiency can easily affect the whole body, unbalancing the entire metabolic network and causing illness.

Taking it a step further, if a nutritional deficiency can cause this, then supplementing the body with the missing nutrients can cure it. The powders, capsules or tablets of free-form amino acids are perhaps the most effective nutritional supplements available today. 'Free-form' means they are separated from the long protein chains in which they naturally occur. The tremendous advantage of taking them in their free-form rather than as protein is that they bypass the need for digestion and are instead absorbed straight through the gut wall. One of the great problems of amino acid deficiency is that it blocks the production of digestive enzymes. The result is to prevent the amino acids contained in the protein you eat from being released. Instead they sit in the gut and feed bacteria. The resulting putrefaction releases other dangerous substances, making the domino effect radiate ever more wildly. As they don't need enzymes to digest them, free-form amino acids are unaffected. Taking amino acids is like spring-loading each domino – you stop it from ever falling down.

Now that you understand how amino acids can help you, how do you know which ones to take for particular illnesses and disorders? On the one hand, it's enormously encouraging that health food shops stock an ever-growing selection of these extraordinary substances, on the other, most aminos have long, bewildering names and their containers give almost no indication of how you should use them and for what. So before going on to the main body of the book – seeing in detail how they work to relieve a variety of ailments – what follows is a short introduction to each amino acid in turn.

Ground rules

Strangely, there is no hard and fast rule about how many amino acids there are. Some people say eight; others say twelve, and many insist on eighteen, twenty-two, and even twenty-five. We'll be looking at twenty aminos in particular – those which have been found most effective in relieving a variety of health disorders. Of these it's generally agreed that only eight cannot be made by the body. Because of this they are called the essential amino acids. They are: **Phenylalanine, Tryptophan, Methionine, Lysine, Leucine, Isoleucine, Valine** and **Threonine**. From these the body can, if necessary, use metabolic pathways to synthesize all the others. These are called non-essential amino acids and include: **Tyrosine, Asparagine, Aspartic acid, Serine, Cysteine, Arginine, Ornithine, Histidine, Glutamic acid, Glutamine, Proline** and **Glycine**. It's always preferable to obtain all non-essential aminos from your diet as manufacturing them in the body might divert the eight essential amino acids from meeting other needs. Don't worry if their names mean nothing to you at the moment. Many of them will be appearing frequently in these pages and you'll soon be able to recognize their highly individual metabolic 'personalities'.

Essential Amino Acids

Phenylalanine

Phenylalanine is considered an essential dietary amino acid. Normally it can't be made by the body from other amino components so we must obtain what we need from our food. Good sources of phenylalanine include beef, chicken, fish, soy, eggs, cottage cheese and milk. Phenylalanine has several important roles in the body's metabolism. As soon as it is digested and absorbed into the liver a certain amount is used to build the sugar-regulating hormone insulin and other proteins and enzymes. It also contributes to a variety of fibrous protein structures, including collagen and elastin.

The remaining phenylalanine acts as the parent molecule of one of the most important metabolic pathways in your body – a pathway that produces brain chemicals called catecholamines –

also known as neurotransmitters. When released from the nerve cells, neurotransmitters cause arousal, an elevated and positive mood and the 'fight or flight' instinct. The best known is the hormone adrenalin. When the pathway is working smoothly these substances allow you to cope with stress. Stress is a continual part of our lives and if this pathway becomes blocked the stress you encounter may quickly overcome you, leading to anxiety and depression and later to serious physical illness. So keeping this pathway supplied with phenylalanine, is immensely important. Phenylalanine can rouse depression victims, protect women from the emotionally draining effects of pre-menstrual tension and has even been found to improve learning potential.

As it is so important we'll be examining every stage of the phenylalanine-adrenalin pathway in chapter 5. For the time being, however, let's look for a moment at the first stage. This sees an enzyme called phenylalanine hydroxylase convert phenylalanine to another amino acid called tyrosine. A small number of people suffer from a disease which causes a deficiency of this conversion enzyme. The disease is called phenylketonuria (better known as PKU) and as it leads to a build-up of phenylalanine it means that there is insufficient tyrosine for the production of the neurotransmitters (catecholamines). Another result is that the work rate of the thyroid gland slows down. The thyroid gland is responsible for the rate of your body's metabolism. It determines how fast you grow, whether the food you eat is stored as fat, burnt as energy or used in the processes of regeneration. It does all this by secreting a regulatory hormone called thyroxin. The amino acid component of this hormone is tyrosine. Phenylketonuria prevents adequate tyrosine reaching the thyroid gland. The results can be fatigue, obesity, lack of growth, and reduced resistance to disease. All this can be avoided by supplementing your diet with tyrosine together with the mineral co-factor iodine.

Few people suffer from phenylketonuria but even so, supplementing the metabolic pathways with free-form supplements of tyrosine as well as phenylalanine can improve your health dramatically. By stimulating the thyroid gland, for instance the increased rate of metabolism – mobilizing the fat deposits – can help you to lose weight. As another of phenylalanine's pathways produces a hormone which curbs appetite it makes the two aminos particularly helpful when included in a weight-loss programme. As they improve your body's production of adrenalin you should not take them if you suffer from high blood pressure. The other side of this coin is that people suffering from low blood pressure benefit enormously from using them.

We mentioned earlier that most amino acids are taken solely in their 'L' forms. Phenylalanine can also be taken in its 'D' form (usually the two are taken in a blend called DLPA). In this state it is a powerful pain-killer – especially when used for chronic states such as colitis, rheumatism and migraine.

Tryptophan

Like phenylalanine, tryptophan is an essential amino acid present in most good protein foods such as beef, eggs and nuts (although in much smaller quantities than phenylalanine). Tryptophan was first mentioned as a health aid in 1913 when researchers established a link between the distressing mental illness pellagra and a deficiency of tryptophan. At the time these results were contradicted by a second group of researchers who showed that the disease could be treated with equal success by yeast preparations containing no tryptophan at all. It took more than thirty years for experts to realize that the chemical which relieved pellagra was niacin (vitamin B3). Niacin can be obtained from sources like yeast, which is why it was found to relieve pellagra. But it can also be manufactured in a metabolic pathway which starts with the amino acid tryptophan. Tryptophan's relationship with B vitamins goes beyond this. It also needs vitamin B6 before it can be metabolized effectively. You may remember in the previous chapter that depriving tryptophan of B6 causes it to be excreted in the urine as xanthurenic acid. Urinary screenings which pick this up not only prove that the body is wasting tryptophan, but also point to low levels of the converting chemical, vitamin B6.

So what are tryptophan's main uses? First, as we have seen, it will ensure that adequate amounts of B3 are manufactured if this vitamin is in short supply. As even minor B3 deficiencies can lead to psychotic disorders; tryptophan helps to avoid this. Most interest, however, lies in tryptophan's relationship with the neuro-transmitter serotonin. This substance is involved in blood clotting and the flushing and dilating effects of the immune response. More importantly, serotonin works both as an inhibitory and excitory neurotransmitter, depending on its concentration in the nervous system. For most people, serotonin calms the brain in much the same way as noradrenalin and adrenalin excite. This is not to say that serotonin leads to depression. Far from it. As depression is often the result of an overactive mind the soothing affects of serotonin actively work to relieve it. Used either in conjunction with phenylalanine or by itself, tryptophan – as the precursor of serotonin – is a natural and harmless alternative to the dangerous antidepressant drugs. Drugs, after all, are substances which are foreign to your body's chemistry. They force a response. Foods, like amino acids, provide natural substances which allow a normal response to occur.

Serotonin is also the substance your brain releases to bring about sleep. Tryptophan, therefore, makes a sounder alternative to sleeping pills if you suffer from insomnia. Furthermore, as it works by enhancing a natural metabolic pathway you won't suffer from any drowsy side-effects the following day; during normal waking hours the body secretes an enzyme which deactivates the sleep-inducing effects.

Tryptophan is used to relieve some migraines. This ability, too, can be attributed to its serotonin-producing pathway and the dilatory effect it has on blood vessels – relieving the pressure areas which cause migraine by distributing the blood more widely. Tryptophan also encourages the production of antibodies, thereby strengthening your immune system against infection and disease.

Sulphur-based aminos

All the aminos we've looked at so far, although important for your physical wellbeing are particularly notable, in free-form supplements, for their effects on the brain. They banish depression, increase alertness, assist sleep and so on. The next group of aminos work by improving the state of your body tissue. These are the sulphur-based amino acids.

The mineral sulphur is a vitally important nutrient for our bodies. It protects the cells from airborne pollutants such as car and aeroplane exhaust, and factory smoke. It slows down the ageing process in the cells and encourages the efficient production of protein. We need sulphur for healthy skin, bones, organs and hair. It helps to transport important elements around the body such as selenium and zinc, and sulphur compounds have even been found to protect the body against radiation. Every day we use up or excrete a total of 850 mg. Yet even eggs, one of the richest sources of sulphur, contain only about 65 mg each. To compensate nature has supplied us with the sulphur-based amino acids – **methionine, taurine, cysteine** and **cystine**. By incorporating these aminos into the huge protein chains, sulphur atoms, which are clamped to the carbon skeletons along with the other constituent atoms, can be stored in the body in large amounts. One gramme of free-form cystine, for example, provides 180 mg of sulphur – nearly three times the amount contained in one egg.

Only one of these four aminos, methionine, is a dietary essential. Methionine is found in dairy products and meat, but is low in most vegetables and legumes. Vegetarians might need to supplement their normal diets with methionine. As a sulphur-based amino, it improves the tone and pliability of skin and conditions the hair. It strengthens nails that are soft and suffer from easy splitting. And it relieves joint pains caused by sulphur deficiency in the connective tissue.

Methionine is a chelator, which means that it locates damaging heavy metals such as lead, cadmium and mercury, then literally grabs on to them, eliminating them from the body like a bouncer throwing an unwelcome drunk into the street. As these metals can lead to hyperactivity, skin complaints, emphysema, diseases and premature ageing methionine can be regarded as a most important part of out diets.

As we have already seen (p. 15) methionine is also the main component of the chemical s-adenosyl-methionine. This substance is used widely in the metabolic pathways to give one nutrient the molecule it needs to become another. When you realize that noradrenalin needs to react with this methionine-based chemical before it can become adrenalin you begin to see the way that amino acids react with each other in the body. This interdependence – the action of one substance working to strengthen the action of another – is known as synergy. It is one of the reasons for the success of free-form amino acids when they are used in nutritional counselling.

The other three sulphur-based aminos can, if necessary – and if the vitamin and mineral co-factors are present – be manufactured in the body from methionine. However, as this diverts the existing methionine from its own duties, such as converting adrenalin, it's much better to use supplements. But what do these three aminos do? In the body cysteine will readily convert to cystine and vice versa, so for the sake of convenience from now on we'll refer to either as cysteine. Like methionine cysteine is a chelator. It eliminates heavy metals and could well have a use in arthritis prevention. It also protects the body from the poisonous effects of alcohol, preventing hangovers, brain and liver damage and emphysema. And it is used by some nutritionists to break down the mucus deposits of diseases such as bronchitis and cystic fibrosis.

Finally, taurine is one of the most abundant amino acids in the body. It is especially common in the excitable tissues of the central nervous system, where it is thought to have a regulating influence. Taurine supplements have been found to control motor tics, such as facial twitches, as well as epileptic seizures. It is also used to relieve angina.

27

The one drawback of these sulphur-based aminos is that in powder form they have a ghastly, rotten-egg odour and taste. This is a case where, unless you have superb self-control or no taste buds, it's wiser to chose the pill or capsule form rather than the powder.

Lysine

Lysine is another dietary essential amino acid which, like methionine, is deficient in vegetables and, especially, in grains, seeds and nuts. One way in which the body uses lysine is as a carrier molecule for calcium, ensuring that adequate amounts are absorbed in the gut and distributed to wherever they are needed. Lysine is also required in the formation of collagen, the latticework-like tissue that makes up much of your body. It is present in bone, cartilage and connective tissue.

Lysine also combines with methionine to produce another amino acid called **Carnitine**. This amino plays a vital role in the body, carrying fatty acids into the cells where they are burnt to release energy. Carnitine helps to prevent heart disease and is a valuable aid in weight reduction programmes.

One particularly interesting use of lysine is its application in cases of herpes (see chapter 11). Briefly, tests have shown that it suppresses the virus in over 90 per cent of those victims who used it. Many are delighted to experience a complete remission. In nearly everyone who uses it their pain disappears overnight and the resolution of existing vesicles is much more rapid than usual.

Branched chain aminos

The branched-chain amino acids (BCAAs) are a group of three essential aminos – **Leucine, Isoleucine** and **Valine** – which are used in the muscles. They are found in nuts and seeds and a good balance of these three aids wound-healing and helps to build up muscle.

Non-essential Amino Acids

Arginine

Since we've mentioned lysine's connection with herpes, we must now bring in the amino acid **Arginine**. While lysine suppresses the herpes virus arginine has been found actually to encourage it.

Therefore when using amino therapy to fight herpes it's important to keep the lysine: arginine ratio high in lysine's favour. One way you can do this is to take the amino acid **L-ornithine** instead of arginine. Ornithine is produced by the first conversion stage of one of arginine's chief metabolic pathways. It is as effective as arginine in stimulating the immune system – one of its main roles in the body – yet it has no aggravating effect on the virus. Apart from its relationship with herpes, arginine is one of the most beneficial aminos you can take. Although it is considered non-essential, the body can't manufacture it quickly enough to meet all its needs. Arginine is indispensible for optimum growth. It is most highly concentrated in the skin and connective tissue and following any sort of wounding there is always a need for additional arginine to enable the body to repair itself properly. Nutritionists have found that arginine supplements substantially increase the rate of wound-healing.

Arginine also stimulates the pituitary gland into producing growth hormone. This not only speeds wound-healing it ensures that fat is burnt more efficiently, at the same time building up muscle tissue. It makes arginine a central part of any weight-reducing programme. Many athletes, recognizing how arginine can improve their performance and physiques, include it in their training programmes. Some people have confused arginine with synthetic growth hormones such as anabolic steroids. There is no connection at all. Arginine works simply by encouraging your body to manufacture its own growth hormones. Anabolic steroids can have an adverse effect on many of the body's metabolic pathways.

Finally, there are many reports suggesting that arginine supplements increase sperm count and sperm mobility. The high concentration of arginine in seminal fluid confirms this need for arginine and research shows that an arginine-deficient diet leads to atrophy of the testicles.

Histidine

This amino acid, found particularly in cereals, sits uncertainly on the borderline between a dietary essential and non-essential. Experts are unsure whether it can be manufactured in the body. A histidine imbalance will result in psychological disorders such as anxiety and schizophrenia as well as lethargy and fatigue, a poor appetite and nausea, particularly if the victim is pregnant. This is because histidine is the parent molecule of an important and highly active chemical called histamine. One of histamine's many roles in the body is to act as an inhibitory neurotransmitter. It is used to strengthen the soothing alpha-wave activity of the brain. In the relaxed state which histamine induces a person is much more resistant to anxiety and stress, able to take life 'in their stride'. If you are histidine-deficient the lack of histamine unbalances these neutral alpha rhythms in the brain, allowing the excitory beta waves – responsible for the brain activity which leads to anger and tension – to dominate. Histidine supplements help to prevent this.

Histidine is also part of your immune response, stored as it is in the highly sensitive mast cells. When the cellular damage caused by viruses, toxins or allergens affects a mast cell it bursts to release the histamine. Histamine has a dilatory effect in the blood vessels and this causes the typical swelling, reddening and flushing of the skin (which is why anti-inflammatory drugs are called anti-histamines). Histidine regulates the ratio of helper to suppressor antibody cells. This, together with the fact that it is an excellent chelator makes it one of the best available treatments for auto-immune diseases such as allergies and rheumatoid arthritis. Histidine also improves digestion by increasing the production of stomach acid, treat ulcers and relieves heartburn and the nausea resulting from pregnancy. Since the dilatory action of histamine works to relieve blood pressure it is also used to treat heart disease patients.

Arguably however, its most important role today is in sex therapy. Research shows that the release of histamine from the mast cells is closely related to orgasm. Women who are unable to achieve orgasm are usually low in histamine and greatly benefit from taking supplements of the precursor amino histidine. The problem of premature ejaculation, on the other hand, is attributed to excess histamine and, in another example of synergy, can be regulated by using methionine and calcium (see chapter 9).

Glutamic Acid

This is the most prominent amino acid in wheat. It is involved in the metabolism of sugars and fats. It combines with poisonous ammonia in the brain to produce glutamine – a brain fuel which affects brain functions, improving alertness and mood. Glutamic acid does not seem to be a neurotransmitter itself but can produce gamma-aminobutyric acid (GABA for short) which is an inhibitory neurotransmitter – that is, it has a calming effect. Glutamic acid has already been proved valuable in treating mentally retarded patients and victims of epilepsy. It is used by many people simply as a pick-me-up (see chapter 4). Since it also helps to raise blood sugar levels it is used to treat hypoglycematics (victims of low blood sugar). It has also been found to stifle the cravings that many people have for alcohol and sweets.

These are the most important and regularly used amino acids. Others which we'll occasionally meet include **asparagine** which can be used in mental and emotional disorders, **glutathione**, a tripeptide (see p. 112 for explanation) which prevents free radical activity, and **glycine** which inhibits activity in the spinal chord.

In this chapter we've seen how one amino acid guards against toxicity, another works as a tranquillizer, and a third can improve sexual activity. Yet this only gives the barest glimpse of the real health potential of amino acids. The skill comes in using them together. Although many people have found relief by taking them individually, amino acids work best when they can react in the body with their complementary amino acids. For example, in a later chapter we'll see a formula for relieving anxiety that includes a blend of four aminos – histidine, tryptophan, glycine and taurine. The different ways in which these aminos affect the body create a synergistic overlap. Unlike drugs of single-strand nutritional support, the effects of such a blend are much greater than the sum of its parts.

Knowing which aminos to include in a blend is the most skilful, and most satisfying, part of amino therapy. In each chapter throughout the book we'll be looking at complex medical problems, seeing which metabolic pathways are affected, then suggesting what we believe to be the best possible blend that you can take to relieve them. It means that you can effectively use these against anything from alcoholism and smoking to allergies, viruses, skin complaints, and sexual problems. As well as listing assorted combinations of aminos, we'll be including vitamins and minerals. These are vital in ensuring that the aminos are fully metabolized by the body. If you like, think of co-factors as the metabolic cement to the amino acids' building blocks.

Now that we're familiar with the basic roles that amino acids play in the body, and their potential for enhancing health, it's time to see how they work in practice. In Part Two, we'll look at the various applications of amino acids for modifying behaviour and relieving mood disorders. We'll see how they can be used to combat stress, dispel anxiety and depression and even enhance memory. To understand how they do this means taking a close look at the way they affect the most complex organ of all – the brain.

Aminos and the body

Lysine
Helps to combat herpes.

Arginine and Ornithine
Can increase sperm count, strengthen immune system and stimulate growth hormone secretion to aid muscle growth and fat metabolism.

Histidine
Precursor of histamine a strong vasodilator. Has a calming effect on anxiety victims (and relieves symptoms such as nailbiting). It also helps to relieve frigidity in women and hastens orgasm in men.

Cysteine and Methionine
Natural chelators of heavy metal. These sulphur-based aminos, promote healthy, supple skin. Methionine also helps reduce liver fat and protects the kidneys.

Glycine
Functions as an inhibitory neuro-transmitter in the nervous system. Together with **Taurine** it helps to relieve motor diseases such as spasticity.

Phenylalanine
Precursor of Tyrosine and the excitory catecholomine neurotransmitters and skin pigment, melanin.

Branched chain aminos (Leucine Isoleucine Valine)
Important for muscle growth and repair. Alcoholics and drug addicts are often deficient in leucine.

Tyrosine
With phenylalamine precursor of the catecholamines as well as being important for the manufacture of thyroxin, a hormone which is vital in regulating the body's rate of growth and metabolism.

Tryptophan
Deficiency causes insomnia and depression. Precursor of vitamin B3.

PART TWO

AMINO BRAIN POWER

Chapter 4

The Matter of Mind and Memory

Nowhere is the potential of amino acids for improving health greater than in the way they assist brain metabolism. The brain is the master control centre of your whole body. It determines every metabolic function and therefore its power is awesome. The best way to come to terms with the sheer ability of your brain is to think of it as an enormous reference library. All you have to do is to substitute a collection of well-thumbed books for a mass of highly sensitive and chemically active cells. For in the same way that the encyclopedias and textbooks of a reference library house reams upon reams of wisdom and learning, so the brain cells are a great storehouse of priceless information which the body must have in order to live. It's when something happens to block the distribution of this information that illness, mental and physical, results.

Your brain receives thousands of requests a second to supply some piece of information from its cells. They come in the form of messages which are brought by the nervous system from every point in the body. It's the brain's job to sort through these messages – matching and comparing them with the mass of knowledge which it has accumulated through a lifetime of experiences – and find an appropriate response to each of them. If, for example, a message comes from the stomach saying that it contains freshly eaten food the brain searches through its reference library of cells until it discovers how it responded to a similar message in the past. Then, having found a precedent, it sends out a reply ordering the stomach to secrete the digestive acids and enzymes.

Of course, these orders are as varied as the needs of your body. There are commands for muscles to contract, for the heart to pump faster, orders to go to sleep or alternatively to get excited. Whatever the message, it must be despatched from the brain as quickly as the request for information arrives. For example, the time it takes for the bang of a burst paper bag to be received by the brain as a nerve message and the order sent out to the body to give a start is approximately one thirtieth of a second. We began by calling the brain a reference library. However, a librarian would never be given the job of cross-referencing it. There are over six billion nerve cells in the brain (half the total amount for the whole body) and each one shares the information which determines its response with up to ten thousand others. The poor librarian would have to compile an index containing a quadrillion entries.

This fantastic interconnection is what gives the brain its versatility. With it the brain can run the millions of subconscious reactions that occur daily, as well as providing the conscious functions of memory, inquisitiveness, reason and emotion. In truth, nothing in your body will work if the brain doesn't. It determines not only emotional and mental states but also the energy levels, growth and general health and functioning of the body. Many of the body's most unpleasant illnesses, including Parkinson's disease, Alzheimer's disease, senility and schizophrenia, are caused as a direct result of brain dysfunction.

Now, thanks to today's metabolic approach to nutrition, neither these, nor other brain problems such as manic depression and anxiety, have to be accepted as an inevitable part of many people's lives. Because by understanding the relationship between nutrition and your brain chemistry, then by using amino acids, their vitamin co-factors and mineral activators to supplement your diet there are few limits to what can be accomplished. Man is a biochemical being whose biochemistry can be influenced nutritionally – for better or worse. And brain changes are not the simple accidents of nature which many people believe.

The connective mechanism of your brain – the way that one cell passes information to, and receives information from, the next – is the important element in learning to use amino acid brain therapy. Let's see how these connections work.

Good Connections

When a message is carried by the nervous system, either into the brain or back to the part of the body waiting for orders, it is transmitted through the nerve cells as an electrical wave. This wave is conducted through one cell at a time, passing to the tip of a branch-like structure on the cell's surface called an axon. From here the message is transmitted from the axon across the minute space which separates one cell from another – a synapse – to a receiving branch on the neighbouring cell called a dendrite. The message then passes through this second cell to its own axon before crossing to the dendrite of a third cell. The relaying process continues until the message reaches its destination.

What interests us most, though, is the way the message travels across the synapse. It's tempting to think of this passage from axon to dendrite as resembling the action of a sparking plug in a car, the electrical wave bridging the gap on its own. In fact, it doesn't happen like this at all. The wave is unable to cross this space and depends instead on a special chemical to carry it. This chemical is contained in a sac at the tip of the axon. The sac bursts as it is contacted by the electrical wave, releasing the chemical into the synapse to make contact with the adjacent cell's dendrite. This contact between chemical and dendrite triggers an electrical wave in the second cell, which passes through to the axon on the cell's far side, activating the release of another messenger chemical, and so on. After use the chemical is either deactivated by enzymes or reabsorbed into the sac.

So you can see that nerve fibres are far from the simple conducting cables that most people imagine. They are, in fact, a series of relay stations that depend on special chemicals every bit as much as they do on electrical impulses. A different chemical exists for each type of message, but collectively they are called neurotransmitters. In 1950 only five neurotransmitters had been discovered; today the number is forty and scientists believe that there may be many more waiting to be found. Every message to and from the brain needs these substances. Some affect our emotions, allowing us to feel happy or angry; others enable us to move, contracting and relaxing muscles. Often many messages are carried at once, such as for sexual arousal. When we take a mind-altering drug, whether it be a sleeping pill, an anti-depressant, alcohol or LSD, it works either by altering the chemical composition of the neurotransmitters themselves or their receptors sites.

Crucially, almost all these neurotransmitters are made from amino acids. There is strong evidence to show that many of the most important neurotransmitters – such as adrenalin and serotonin – are directly diet-dependent. In other words, the levels of these substances in the brain, and therefore the way your brain works, can be directly influenced by what you eat. So, by using free-form amino supplements in your diet to manipulate the levels of the particular amino acids which make up the neurotransmitters, the nature and intensity of the brain messages they carry can actually be altered. Many mood disorders such as depression and anxiety, which can both lead to physical illness, are inextricably linked with deficiencies of certain neurotransmitters. For example, your brain wouldn't be able to produce all the adrenalin it needs to help you respond to stress if your body didn't have enough of the parent aminos phenylalanine and tyrosine. The results would be torpor, lethargy and depression. But, by providing your body with a free-form supplement of extra phenylalanine you can actually relieve the problem.

We'll see exactly how this approach works in the following three chapters when we look at some brain-related disorders in depth. And we'll suggest blends of amino acids, with their vitamin and mineral co-factors, which have been found to give the greatest relief from problems such as stress, chronic depression and anxiety neurosis. For the moment, though, let's take a look at some amino acids which you may find helpful even if you enjoy a healthy mental and emotional state. We've all suffered at times from not being as alert as we'd like, from days when we've found it impossible to concentrate, and even from forgetfulness. Amino acids can help with these problems too.

Amino Brain Booster

One of the most highly successful free-form amino supplements for helping to maintain efficient brain functions is glutamic acid. As it can be manufactured in the body from other amino acids, glutamic acid is considered to be a dietary non-essential and until recently many experts thought that it provided very little nutritional benefit. Now more and more people are recognizing its importance to the brain. Like most aminos, glutamic acid is used in several different metabolic pathways; one is of particular interest to us here.

Glutamic acid is necessary for ridding the brain of ammonia – one of nature's most highly poisonous chemicals. If allowed to accumulate in the body ammonia causes irritability, nausea, vomiting, tremors, hallucinations and eventually death. Unfortunately, this toxin is created by the disposal of worn-out protein, a natural consequence of the body's metabolism. This continuous process occurs when the amino group and the acid group are split off from the spent protein molecule. While they provide energy for the body, the leftover nitrogen, which has no energy value at all, is left to accumulate as ammonia. Therefore, wherever amino acids are used – and that means everywhere in the body – ammonia is certain to be present.

The process your body employs to clear the ammonia is called the urea cycle – a metabolic pathway which converts ammonia to urea. In this form the body can harmlessly excrete ammonia in its urine. And this is where glutamic acid comes in. Because the first and most important stage of the urea cycle is the reaction of glutamic acid with ammonia. The two combine to produce the harmless chemical glutamine. But if your body doesn't have enough glutamic acid to convert all the ammonia the toxicity levels will rise very quickly.

The implications of this for the brain are frightening. As 25 per cent of all the body's metabolic activity occurs in the brain, even when the urea cycle is working perfectly the waste product of its metabolic activity, ammonia, will be much more concentrated than anywhere else. When a shortage of glutamic acid allows the ammonia levels to rise even slightly the results include fatigue, confusion and an inability to concentrate, as well as exaggerated mood swings. So you can see how important it is to make sure that your body has an ample supply of glutamic acid at all times.

By using ammonia in its transformation, glutamic acid helps to detoxify the brain of this potentially lethal chemical. There is, however, one problem in supplementing your brain's normal supplies of glutamic acid. Scientists have found that it doesn't easily cross the blood brain barrier, a membraneous substance which protects the brain cells from the poisons carried in the blood. Glutamine, on the other hand, crosses with ease. Once in the brain it will convert to glutamic acid before combining with ammonia and converting back to glutamine. This is why many nutritionists will recommend that you take glutamine rather than glutamic acid.

In a pamphlet on glutamine (see References, p. 199) the biochemist Richard Passwater says that this amino, like the sugar glucose, can also be used by the brain as a source of energy. Finally, glutamic acid is also a necessary component of one of the B vitamins, folic acid. Many nutritionists have cited folic acid deficiency as a cause of irritability, forgetfulness and general mental sluggishness.

Taking glutamine is almost like plugging your brain into a free energy source. Not only does it make you feel healthier, it can also benefit your work. Students, for example, have found that glutamine supplements taken in the evening help them to concentrate on homework and revision. They can also work much later into the night without feeling tired. Unlike the caffeine contained in tea and coffee, glutamine stimulates the brain by naturally supporting the brain's metabolic pathways. You feel livelier when you take glutamine because it unblocks the vitality we all possess but rarely exploit; coffee provides an artificial arousal at the expense of your health. Students have also taken glutamine before sitting examinations. They report greater mental alertness and clarity and few of the worrying doubts that often result from the pressure of exams.

Glutamine is one of the amino acids widely used in the USA to combat jetlag. It allows you to travel comfortably for long periods without needing to sleep so that you can adapt much more quickly to local time.

Businessmen are also discovering how helpful glutamine can be.

John works in the foreign exchange offices of a multinational bank in the City. He spends most of his day on the the phone, buying and selling large amounts of currency. Before transactions he trawls for information, warily interpreting the 'mood' of the international money markets. He has to be sensitive to every price fluctuation and trend, with thousands of dollars resting on the outcome of his decisions. It's a highly stressful job.

When he came for nutritional counselling he complained of extreme tiredness at work: 'It's as if I knew what I had to do but just couldn't engage my brain,' he recalled. 'My mind was active in a way that a fly is active when it's stuck to fly-paper – all that expenditure of energy with no result. I was getting less and less done and making some pretty bad decisions. Half the time I couldn't care less, the other half I was panic-stricken. John was advised to take 250 mg of glutamine three times a day, together with 400 mcg of the complementary folic acid, 100 mg of vitamin B6 and 500 mg of vitamin C. The surge in his energy and enthusiasm for work took place overnight. 'I felt so refreshed,' he said. 'It was as if I was in a state of constantly having just stepped out of an invigorating shower.'

Memories Are Made Of This

Another common and annoying problem is loss of memory. How often have you seen a face and been unable to put a name to it, or tried in vain to remember a word you wanted to use or the title of a film you once saw? Have you ever left on a trip only to freeze in horror when you couldn't remember whether you'd turned the oven off or closed a window? For most of us this forgetfulness is only a minor frustration. For some it is deadly serious. The chronic forms of memory loss are presenile (occurring before sixty years of age) and senile (occurring after sixty) dementia. In their acute stages they leave victims with little awareness of who they are or of their surroundings, unresponsive to those around them and often incontinent. Now, as a result of research conducted into the severest forms of this distressing illness, amino acids are being used to help not only these but also the milder forms of memory loss which we all experience.

Much of this important research was conducted in the 60s and 70s by doctor Carl Pfeiffer at his Brain Bio Centre in Princeton. Pfeiffer started by challenging traditionally held views about the causes of senility. Up until then, physicians believed that the blame for this illness lay mainly with arterioschlerosis, the loss of pliability and hardening of blood vessels with its resulting build-up of fatty plaques in the brain. The theory is that the arteriosclerosis strangles the blood vessels, starves the brain cells of nutrients and causes brain damage. After conducting tests on a group of patients all suffering from senility, Pfeiffer was forced to disagree with this view. Only a third of these patients actually had arteriosclerosis. While he wouldn't deny that this was indeed one of the causes of senility, there were obviously other, perhaps more direct, causes too.

Carrying these tests further, he eventually found that the one factor which all these patients had in common was low levels of spermine in the blood and brain. Spermine is a product of the amino acid arginine and found in semen, blood tissue and brain cells. When Pfeiffer examined the spermine levels of people with good memories he found their levels to be many times higher than those of the senility victims. It seems fairly certain that when your body has low levels of spermine your memory is badly effected.

The theory put forward to explain how spermine deficiency impairs memory is quite complicated. It goes back to the production of ribonucleic acid (RNA). You may remember that the body uses RNA to duplicate sections of the master blueprint – DNA – whenever tissue needs to be repaired or to grow. The RNA copy is used to select the number and assortment of substances that are needed to make the particular section of tissue. However, in the brain cells it seems that RNA is also important for storing our memories.

RNA is made by an enzyme RNA polymerase. And this enzyme is activated by spermine. Insufficient spermine in your body will lead to a deficiency of brain RNA, in turn causing a loss of memory. Therefore, raising spermine levels increases the production of RNA and actually helps to improve your memory. Spermine is produced from arginine by a complicated metabolic pathway involving several co-factors. All these nutrients must be included in any memory-enhancing formula, so let's look at the pathway to see how it works. It starts when arginine reacts with an enzyme activated by manganese to produce the amino acid ornithine. Reacting in turn with vitamin B6, ornithine is converted to another substance called putrescine. At this point 'activated' methionine – itself created from magnesium and methionine – converts putrescine first to spermidine and then to spermine.

From time to time we'll be giving you lists of aminos (together with vitamin and mineral co-factors) which we suggest you take in a blend. These lists are specifically formulated to relieve particular disorders and each nutrient is included for the way it enhances the potency of the others. We've decided for the most part to leave

41

decisions about quantities to you – one person's metabolism varies so much from another's that it would be impossible to decide on amounts that suited everyone. As a rule you might try between 250 mg and 1500 mg of each amino a day, starting on the low side and gradually building up if at first you find no relief. As for the vitamins and minerals the best thing to do here is simply follow the directions on their labels.

Therefore, if you want to help the arginine to spermine pathway to progress smoothly – and so improve your memory – try a blend of the following aminos and co-factors, taken once or twice a day between meals:

Aminos

methionine
arginine
ornithine

Co-factors

B6
vitamin C
manganese
magnesium

Perhaps when you're confronted with a list like this, and imagine the small mountain of supplements you might have to wade through, you feel tempted to stick with the convenient bottle of pills prescribed by your doctor. Don't be. Like most worthwhile things amino supplementation involves a little bit of work and application. Once you decide which aminos and co-factors are best for you stick to that decision and take them regularly. It can be so easy to miss a dosage or two that before long, you'll have stopped taking them altogether. Try not to do this. Amino-based nutritional therapy is one of the most effective, and thorough, forms of health treatment you can use. If you stick with amino acids and their vitamin and mineral complementaries they will pay you dividends in terms of your health and vitality.

Aminos and the brain

Cerebral cortex

Arginine
As the precursor of spermidine and spermine it helps to improve memory

Histidine
Although present in concentrations only one tenth those of noradrenalin or serotonin, histidine (as the precursor of histamine) has a powerful calming effect as it promotes tranquil alpha wave activity

Pituitary gland

GABA (Gamma Amino Butyric Acid)
An inhibitory neurotransmitter it slows down the neuron firing rate

Glutamine
Acts as a brain fuel and may be an excitory neurotransmitter. Clears poisonous ammonia from the brain. Aids concentration and reduces mental fatigue

Tryptophan
Precursor of the inhibitory neuro-transmitter, serotonin. This relieves insomnia and combats depression. It is the precursor of B3 which helps to prevent mental disturbances

Phenylalanine & Tyrosine
Precursors of the catech-olamines. These excitory neurotransmitters (nor-adrenalin and adrenalin) are important for easing depressive and stressed behavior

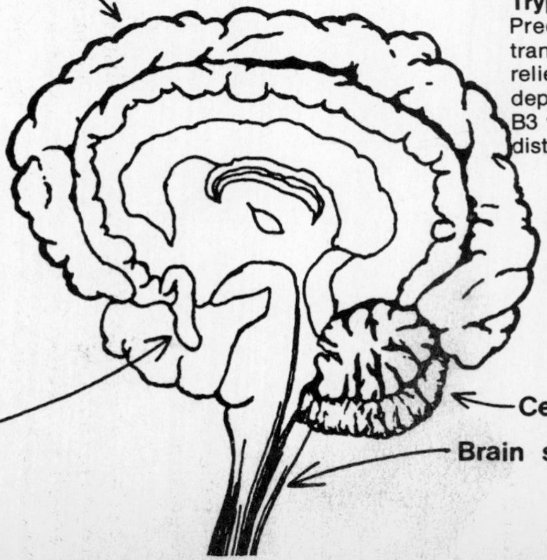

Cerebellum

Brain stem

43

Chapter 5

Stresswatch

By now most people realize that uncontrolled stress brings trouble. It contributes to insomnia, gastric ulcers, high blood pressure, asthma and migraine, for instance. Prolonged or excessive stress is also considered a major factor in premature ageing and the development of degenerative diseases. Stress will strip your body of essential nutrients like a thief in a jeweller's shop. Unfortunately, with the high-pressure demands of our society, continual contact with the factors that cause stress – stressors – is inevitable. What we can do is to use amino acid supplementation to strengthen dramatically the body's ability to cope with stress when it occurs.

But what is stress? A climber clinging uncertainly to the finger-holds on a cliff face feels stress. So does a child waiting for a school bus in the freezing rain or a housewife who burns her hand in the kitchen. Although their specific reactions vary – the climber begins to sweat and gets a tight stomach, a child goes pale and starts to shiver and the housewife suffers from physical inflammation and emotional shock – their internal biochemical responses are working in a stereotyped manner common to all which helps them to cope with the increased demands made upon their bodies. Each undergoes the increased production of corticoid hormones and adrenalin, as well as a number of other biochemical, neurological and physical changes. This is called the stress response; and it takes place in exactly the same way, regardless of what has caused the stress.

Understanding the stress response and the biochemical changes it brings about is important. It will show you how to improve your body's ability to cope with stress by providing it with the necessary support. This in turn can lead to an improvement in health, a balancing of emotions and the prevention of premature ageing and degeneration.

Of course, stress isn't only confined to such extreme physical conditions: it can occur in a thousand different ways. In one form or another stress factors are besieging the body night and day like a massive arsenal bearing down on almost every avenue of life, insidiously affecting your body. Emotions we all experience many times a day such as anger, anxiety, fear or depression are stressors. So are prolonged fatigue, severe physical exhaustion (from work or play) and starvation diets. The self-imposed calorie restriction practised by many slimmers can cause great stress. So can many other occurrences such as allergic reactions to food or environmental factors ranging from house dust and pollen to atmospheric chemicals; infections, whether viral, bacterial or fungal; pre- and post-operative stress associated with surgery; degenerative or chronic debilitative conditions; jetlag and insomnia. Even the minor spasms of anger and frustration felt in a traffic jam or at a train cancellation cause stress. All are so much a part of modern life that we take them for granted.

Stereotypes of Stress

While people's responses to stress are as varied as the number of stressors they encounter, the biological nature of the response is a rigid stereotype. It is called the general adaptation syndrome (GAS) and its purpose is to maintain stability in the body's structure and function – homeostasis – and ultimately, in fact, to preserve life. Every stressor disrupts homeostasis to some extent. When this happens GAS comes into play. It has three stages: alarm, resistance and exhaustion.

During the alarm stage your body's overall resistance to disease is lowered and the sympathetic nervous system fires. This is responsible for our 'fight or flight' instincts. To meet the increased demands the brainwaves change, blood flow is increased to the muscles and adrenalin is secreted more quickly.

With the resistance stage your body's systems are mobilized to meet the threat of the stressor. This stage can last for a long time or a short time, depending on the intensity of your reaction to the threat. The longer it continues, the more of your body's vital nutrients will be depleted in sustaining it.

The body rarely gets to the final stage of GAS. But when it does your weakest systems break down and chronic fatigue and illness follow. If the exhaustion stage continues a person eventually dies – although this usually only happens in cases of extreme shock or with old age.

We can see the kind of biochemical demands that stress makes on the body by looking at the metabolic reactions necessary to sustain the alarm and resistance stages of GAS. This is what happens. Protein is broken down (especially in the muscles) and there is a mobilization of fat and a retention of salt. Minerals such as potassium are lost and in traumatized people there is low liver protein synthesis, impaired kidney function and decreased immune functions, leading to fatigue and susceptibility to illness. These people increase their amino acid consumption to meet the heightened metabolic requirements of stress, amino acids which are needed elsewhere in the metabolic pathway network. Although these examples may seem extreme, they show just the kind of violence that prolonged stress does to the body's natural biochemical balance and wellbeing. Even if our reaction to stress in normal circumstances is only a fraction of this, our metabolic balance is slowly but surely chipped away by the effects of simple, everyday stress. How can we ensure that we are physiologically able to deal with stress year after year without suffering any negative consequences? The answer lies in something called adaptive energy.

To Each His Own

We all react to stress in the same way. Different people find different things stressful, but certain stressors such as injury affect everyone. Each person differs in how much stress they can take before reaching the exhaustion stage. This depends partly on conditioning – to what extent we can become familiar with and at ease with something we at first find stressful – but also on the amount of adaptive energy we have. Adaptive energy is unlike caloric energy, which can be replaced by foods. Instead it is more like a well of vitality from which you can draw when you need it. One person can have a great deal – he may be on the move constantly and able to withstand a lot of stress – while another, when faced with the same stress, quickly reaches the GAS stage of exhaustion.

Early researchers believed that once your supply of adaptive energy was used up as a result of the wear and tear of stress nothing could be done to restore it. Now, thanks to new research, we know this is not so. Adaptive energy – your basic vitality – can be enhanced. It can be strengthened so that the exhaustion stage of GAS can be staved off. The best way of achieving this is by fortifying your body with optimum quantities of the nutrients used up in the stress reaction. And it is not one or two nutrients which are necessary to accomplish this, but a whole family of substances which enable your body to respond well to stress. To understand why, let's look first at how each nutrient is involved in the important biochemical changes which take place in the stress reaction as a whole, from the release of adrenalin to the breakdown of protein in the tissue.

The Biochemical Relay Race

Central to GAS is the secretion of adrenalin, which triggers a number of related responses in the body. Adrenalin is the driving force of the stress reaction, as it is the fuel which powers your body's attempts to rise to the demands being made on it. This important hormone is produced by a chain of biological events – a metabolic pathway – beginning with the parent amino acid phenylalanine. Considering the large number of nutrients that are needed to help the process, it is worth describing the reaction step by step to show how important each one is, as well as illustrating the total dependency they have on each other. (See also the diagram on p 49)

The whole process resembles a relay race. For his team's victory each runner counts on the speed of his predecessor, the smoothness of the baton pass and the state of the track, as well as his own fitness. The finishing line in the case of the stress response is the production of adrenalin, and the starting-gun is fired when the parent amino acid phenylalanine reacts with an enzyme called phenylalanine-4-monooxygenase. This produces the amino acid, tyrosine. Tyrosine is acted upon in turn by the enzyme tyrosine-hydroxylase and becomes L-dopa, another amino acid. At this stage vitamin B6 and phosphorus, acting together as co-factors, convert the L-dopa to dopamine. The complex, house-of-cards nature of the whole process become apparent when you realize that to produce this co-factor requires the presence of magnesium – a substance not even included in the equation.

The next stage is the production of noradrenalin from dopamine and it can only occur when the number of reacting vitamins and minerals is enlarged to include vitamin C and copper. Finally, to convert noradrenalin into adrenalin your body has to call on the enzyme-activated form of the amino, methianine-s-adenosyl-methionine. All the enzymes mentioned here – in fact, all enzymes – are made from amino acids, sometimes with vitamin or minerals hook-ups. So you can begin to see how central the supply of these free-form amino acids is, not only for the body's ability to deal with stress but even for its continued existence.

What this means is that when you are taking nutrients as a biological support mechanism, either for general health or a specific healing process, it is vitally important to focus on the entire family, to consolidate the whole metabolic pathway rather than expecting results from any one nutrient. If a relay team spends all their training time running and neglecting baton passing their performance in the race, regardless of their individual speed, will be uncoordinated and they will lose. So it is with the stress pathway: if even a single nutrient is in low supply the biochemical relay will become sluggish and the body will suffer by losing the adequate amounts of adrenalin that it needs.

The message is simple. When the metabolic relay from phenylalanine is not flowing as it should your body's response to stress is inadequate. This is a widespread phenomenon in the West, as are it symptoms of fatigue, lowered resistance to illness, depression and premature ageing. It can, in effect, remove all the sparkle from your life. That's the bad news. The good news is that simply by supplementing your body with free-form amino acids, vitamins and minerals needed for the stress response, you can often easily and surprisingly alter your whole experience of life and health.

Nutritional Answers to Stress Demands

Giving your body the metabolic support it needs not only heightens your resistance to stress damage, it increases your adaptive energy, improves mental functioning and strengthens overall vitality. Despite the great complexity of interrelated metabolic pathways involved, this is not an overwhelmingly difficult task to perform. In essence, it involves examining these metabolic pathways, noting the particular metabolites involved and supplying them through your diet as part of a wisely chosen programme of nutritional supplementation. The metabolic approach to health based on the orthomolecular view of the body – in which you supply its cells with optimum quantities of nutrients needed for high-level functioning – is really so simple that it is amazing to think that it has been largely overlooked by most nutritionists and physicians. Traditionally, they have emphasized individual nutrients and their specific functions in the body without taking into account their interrelationships with the metabolic pathways in which they are used.

Let's briefly look at the nutrients involved in the specific stress-related metabolic pathways. We can then outline the foundations of a metabolic nutritional programme which is the basis of not only high level health but also of effective holistic amino acid supplementation.

Nutrients, Metabolites and Pathways

The destruction of protein during stress produces increased quantities of ammonia. The body can only get rid of this poison

METABOLIC PATHWAY OF THE STRESS RESPONSE

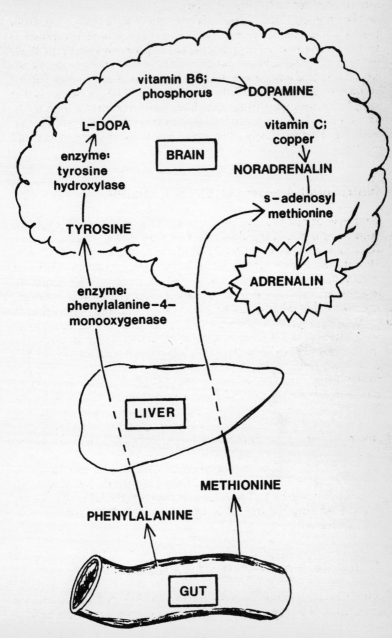

through the urea cycle by consigning the waste into the urine, which is then eliminated from the body. The function of this particular metabolic pathway is maintained thanks to the minerals magnesium and manganese and the vitamins B3 and B6, as well as several amino acids, two of which are particularly helpful when given as supplements – arginine and glutamine.

To support the heavy demands made on the thyroid gland during stress you have to call upon the help of the amino acid tyrosine and the mineral iodine. Combining together in the thyroid, they produce the hormone thyroxin which controls the rate of metabolism not only in the body as a whole but also in individual cells.

The production of the endorphins – the brain's natural opiates – which occurs when the body is under pain-related stress (they are responsible for the runner's high), also need the support of many nutrients. These include phenylalanine, tyrosine, glycine, leucine and methionine. The few athletes who are privy to this knowledge use such a formula to heighten endurance and enhance the bliss that only extreme exertion can bring.

In each of the metabolic pathways involved in stress that have been mentioned, there is a specific collection of nutrients. Although it is not necessary for you to understand all the elaborate biochemical transformations, you can greatly benefit from a general awareness of the nutrients which support them and the relationships between them. They are usually taken three times a day. Used in specific combinations together with a good diet, they can form a foundation for the most powerful antidote to stress known to science. Use them whenever you find yourself under heavy demands from work or emotional worries; if you tend to push your body to its limits in athletics: when recovering from an illness; or any other time when stress – which when you are really healthy is the spice of life – becomes a burden to you.

Aminos
arginine
glutamine
phenylalanine
tyrosine
tryptophan

Co-factors
A
B1
B2

B6
B12
C
E
pantothenic acid
choline
folic acid
niacin
magnesium
potassium
manganese

Chapter 6

Depression – A Brain Symptom

Depression is a paradox: the most spectacularly able thing in the universe – your brain – brought low by an overwhelming sense of futility and uselessness, a belief that life is just too difficult for you to cope with. The brain is the crucible for 25 per cent of all metabolic activity. The six billion nerve cells it contains make up half the total for the whole body. It stimulates motor functions, digestion, growth and tissue repair, interprets our sensory experiences and decides which physical and emotional responses to make. Yet, despite this incredible power, it constitutes only 2 per cent of your body's weight. This makes it highly sensitive. Nutritional deficiencies can cause brain imbalances which send biochemical shockwaves through your entire body; and the emotional wasteground of depression is one of the results. It can be cured. By using free-form amino acids together with their co-factors you can strengthen dramatically the fragile mechanisms of the brain. If you suffer from depression, amino therapy might give you more energy and optimism than you ever realized existed.

Depression is the common cold of mental disorders. One person in a hundred suffers from it right now; if it has never affected you there is a better than one in eight chance that it will. Classic full-blown depression is defined simply as 'the loss of capacity to enjoy life, combined with a poverty of thought and movement'. It's easy enough to glimpse the numbing effects of depression. Picture yourself on a family outing. It's an English summer bank holiday and you're parked in a layby. But the sky is lead grey and sleet spatters horizontally across the windscreen, reducing everyone to a sense of despondency and languor. Conversation is conducted in bad-tempered monosyllables, and even drawing a face on the fogged window requires a huge effort. Despite wanting to drive home, it just doesn't seem to matter enough to bother.

We've all found ourselves in situations like this, senseless of anything but the immediate despondent feelings and blind to the mass of future possibilities. Of course, once the sun comes out we'll remember the frisbee in the boot and the world will be fine. Some people, though, live their lives in this state. This is called pathological depression. It strips the sufferers of their sense of self-worth and leaves them feeling inadequate and unresponsive to the demands of life. Often their mental disorder leads to physical illness, sometimes suicide. Let's examine the specific causes and effects of depression. Then, by seeing which metabolic pathways are involved, we can formulate an amino-based nutritional programme which frees the mind from its smothering grasp.

Anatomy of Depression

Depression has several recognized forms. The first, and most common, variety is called reactive depression. As its name suggests, the victim's depression is a reaction to a stressful event in his life. The death of a loved one is a typical example. This sudden and prolonged stress can quickly deplete your body of vital nutrients, which causes fatigue and torpor. Furthermore, as the death of someone close feels so arbitrary and cruel, it might hardly seem worth making the effort of rousing yourself. After the recent death of his wife, a 67-year-old man slept for six weeks in his living room. This wasn't for sentimental reasons such as the fear of memories that sleeping in his bedroom would bring. The shock of his bereavement simply left him without the energy or mental focus to contemplate climbing the stairs. The same thing could happen if you are made redundant, fail an important exam or separate from your husband or wife.

Endogenous depression is another common form. Unlike reactive depression, it has no obvious cause. Because of this, doctors have difficulty treating it and it often becomes chronic. It is characterized by intense self-hate, apathy, spontaneous crying spells, lack of mental focus and a craving for solitude. And because of the sufferer's indifference to recovery it is often self-perpetuating. Patients sometimes admit to bewilderment when they see others showing enthusiasm for something.

The indifference we feel towards our own well-being when we're in the grip of depression also makes us neglect our diets. The result is widespread nutritional deficiency. The more our bodies are starved of vital nutrients, the greater the demands on the rest of the body become. Before long we are consumed by a widening downward spiral of illness and degeneration.

This is what depression does to us. It is difficult to prevent because its effects may often be delayed or hidden in other symptoms. And it's difficult to treat because once we're in its grip we often don't care whether or not we recover. Acknowledging these facts is one thing; accepting them is quite another. If we can discover where the biochemical imbalances which cause depression occur, we can use amino acids and their co-factors to correct them. Let's start with the most important cells in the body – the nerves.

The Need for Neurotransmitters

You may remember (see chapter 4) how every cell of the nervous system is separated from its neighbour by a small space called a synapse. And that to relay the brain's minute electrical messages from one nerve cell to the next, the nerve endings (axons) must fill the spaces with secretions of neurotransmitters. There are at least forty such conducting chemicals and the metabolic pathways which make them vary with the nature of the messages they carry from the brain. Certain chemicals transmit pain sensations, for example; others cause voluntary muscle movement. Some cause excitory responses; others are inhibitory.

The particular neurotransmitters that govern our excitory emotional responses are the catecholamines, (see the description of the GAS response on pp 46-7) a group derived from the amino acids phenylalanine and tyrosine. In other words, our reactions to everything we encounter in life – the way we are stirred by a piece of music, angered in an argument or amused by a joke – depends on the state of these specific neurotransmitters. Too much or too little of any of these substances will make us underact or overreact, according to the stimuli.

Many psychologists and nutritionists are convinced that depression is caused by deficiencies in the catecholamine group, with poor nutrition or digestion usually to blame. To illustrate the point let's imagine you are under prolonged stress. As long as the sympathetic nervous system operates, the digestion of your food is halted. With this, the protein in the small intestine begins to putrefy, releasing harmful substances like phenylethylamine (PEA) instead of the essential catecholamine parent molecule, phenylalanine. PEA is then absorbed through the intestine wall and circulated in the blood in place of phenylalanine. Far from producing the excitory neurotransmitters, it is converted to octopamine. This is an inactive chemical which takes the place of the catecholamines adrenalin and noradrenalin. Rather than convey the messages from your brain, this chemical imposter blocks them. As a result our reactions, physically and emotionally, become unbalanced. And as adrenalin is the hormone that fires the stress response our bodies are forced to submit to the exhaustion stage of stress. The result: chronic depression.

This spotlights the enormous advantage of free-form amino acids. They don't need to be digested, so there is no danger of putrefaction. They are circulated straight to the affected areas and provide immediate relief.

But if nutrition is important for treating depression why do people so often end up on the psychiatrist's couch? The answer is that until quite recently many people thought that the production of neurotransmitters in the brain occurred independently of the food we ate. This belief was based on the existence of an alignment of protective cells that exists in the brain called the blood brain barrier.

The Blood Brain Border Patrol

One of the many roles of the blood as it travels around the body is to collect the water-soluble toxic wastes from the cells and carry them to the liver and kidneys for excretion. On its journey the blood is pumped through the brain, delivering oxygen and removing carbon dioxide. However, if the toxins that it carries were allowed to come into contact with the highly sensitive brain cells the effects would be catastrophic. Instead, as the blood is channelled into the minute, branched capillaries of the brain, oxygen is filtered out through a sheath of special cells on the capillary wall. At the same time, like xenophobic customs officials, these cells identify the toxins which attempt to enter with the oxygen, and reject them. The toxins must continue to circulate in the blood until reaching the kidneys and liver.

Because the brain is the last organ to suffer when the body starves the blood brain barrier was also thought to protect the brain from any dietary variations. In other words, we could eat as little or as much as we liked without affecting brain functions; the cause of mental disorder was thought to lie elsewhere. We now know this is not true. Whatever we eat directly affects the production of neurotransmitters. And, as neurotransmitters determine our mental and emotional well-being, it follows that when depression occurs we can rectify it nutritionally.

Several amino acids combine to make mood-influencing neurotransmitters. Let's now see how they can be used to provide deep and lasting relief from depression.

DLPA and the PEA-brain

Perhaps the most important and effective amino acid for treating depression is DL-phenylalanine, a combination of two forms. This essential amino is usually prescribed as L-phenylalanine. Most D-form amino acids – mirror-images of L – give no nutritional help and are often converted in the body into their L forms. Phenylalanine is different. Research is showing that D-phenyl-alanine relieves areas of the brain which are unaffected by L. D-phenylalanine on its own is very expensive and nutritionists now prescribe a blend of the two called DLPA. Once the blend reaches the stomach and is broken down, the two forms separate, freeing D-phenylalanine to work on the causes of depression in the brain. Tests have shown it to be between 89 and 100 per cent successful. How does it work?

First, D-phenylalanine (or the DLPA form, but not L-phenylalanine) relieves depression by preventing the breakdown of endorphin hormones. These are the morphine-like substances produced by the adrenal gland along with the catecholamines in times of stress. They are the natural pain-killers which cause the euphoria experienced by athletes as they pass through the 'pain barrier'. Depression victims who have been given endorphins have experienced sudden and dramatic relief. However, to be effective they must be injected either into the spinal column or the brain itself, a dangerous and impractical method. Moreover, they are broken down very quickly by purpose-built enzymes so that any relief is short-lived. D-phenylalanine blocks the action of these enzymes, allowing the antidepressant effects of the endorphins to last much longer. Rather than the body adapting to DLPA and needing progressively more to block the endorphin-destroying enzymes, as it does with antidepressant drugs, the beneficial effects actually accumulate and become stronger with time.

DLPA also strengthens the nerve-cell metabolic pathways which produce the excitory neurotransmitters noradrenalin and adrenalin. They are secreted at those nerve endings which trigger the sympathetic nervous system. If your body can produce enough of these substances to meet its needs it will be much more likely to withstand the mental and emotional stresses that cause depression. If, on the other hand, your cells are depleted – by poor digestion perhaps – they won't be able to 'charge' up the brain when stresses occur.

Catecholamine deficiency was one of the first chemical causes of depression to be pinpointed. Many of today's antidepressant drugs work by stimulating the levels of these substances in the nervous system. Unlike the natural stimulating effects of phenylalanine, however, man-made antidepressants can have serious and harmful side-effects. This is because after stimulating the release of noradrenalin and adrenalin to elevate your mood they stop them from being reabsorbed by the nerve terminals. Instead they are broken down and dispersed, leaving the neurotransmitter levels in the cells depleted. The next time catecholamines are needed the cells are placed under increased stress to yield more without the support of any protein reinforcement. Before long the stores of noradrenalin and adrenalin will be utterly exhausted, resulting in nausea, seizures and anorexia. The advantage of DLPA is that even as it stimulates catecholamine release it strengthens the whole metabolic pathway. The nerve cells are allowed to perform naturally. They reabsorb their neurotransmitters after use, which prevents the harmful deterioration caused by man-made drugs.

Stress Points

The production of noradrenalin is only part of the stress response. As we have seen, the fatigue and disinterest of depression often occur when our bodies are unable to respond to stress demands. Levels of adrenalin are nearly always negligible in depression patients. Providing nutritional support for the entire pathway, therefore, is essential. Together with DLPA you should take the amino acid tyrosine. Tyrosine is a product of phenylalanine and, as it is one step along the metabolic pathway that leads to adrenalin, it encourages the stress response.

The final stage of the pathway, where noradrenalin is converted to adrenalin, needs s-adenosyl-methionine to affect the change. Methionine the precursor of this molecule, also detoxifies the body of histamine. This is important because histamine is an inhibitory neurotransmitter and if it is present in the body in excess it can easily lead to depression. Many victims of chronic depression who, despite following sound nutritional advice, still suffer are often delighted to find that all they needed was a supplement of methionine in their diets.

The importance of stress hormones, the catecholamines, is shown by the case of a patient called Rachel. During the space of ten years she had become progressively more tired and depressed. Finding it hard to exert herself, she eventually decided to give up her job at a firm of management consultants. At home her relationship with her husband seemed equally fruitless, but she simply felt too disinterested to try to change anything. In the face of her almost total unresponsiveness, and seeing no prospect of improvement, her husband left her. 'It was a terrible time,' she said. 'I could always see what needed to be done but there was this massive blanket of inertia holding me back.' Things got worse as she was forced to take a part-time job to support herself and her young son. Conserving all the energy she had for the job, she withdrew completely from any social contact. Luckily for her she decided to come for nutritional counselling. A urinary amino acid test showed that the phenyl-alanine and tyrosine levels in her body were almost non-existent. She was given supplements of these two and their co-factors. There was an immediate improvement. She felt more positive, suddenly found herself full of energy and soon started making plans to renew her life.

A depression victim might try taking this combination of nutrients up to three times a day.

Aminos
DL-phenylalanine
tyrosine
methionine
(One word of caution: no tyrosine or any form of phenylalanine should be taken if you are also taking MAO inhibitors see p. 192.)

Co-factors
magnesium
B1
Zinc
B3
B6
C

As these supplements all work on the same metabolic pathway they create a synergistic overlap – the effects of one treatment complementing the effects of the others. This accounts for the terrific results when they are used to treat depression. Recent double-blind tests (where neither the researchers nor the subjects know who is receiving what) have shown that DLPA is at least as effective as Imipramine, the most commonly prescribed anti-depressant drug, and without any of the harmful side-effects. It is also widely used to relieve the mood disorders associated with pre-menstrual syndrome.

Perchance to Sleep

Once depression is allowed to get hold of you the mental and physical fatigue that result is one of its most unpleasant symptoms. Despite often being near total exhaustion, you will find it impossible to sleep. Lying awake in the small hours, your mind darting anarchically from one thought to another, is a desperate experience. This acute insomnia is caused by a deficiency of the inhibitory neurotransmitter serotonin, the chemical responsible for making us sleep.

As we have seen (p. 15 and p. 25) serotonin's precursor is the active amino acid, tryptophan. But the body also needs tryptophan elsewhere to create vitamin B3. As the nutritional deficiencies of stress and depression compound themselves throughout the body, large amounts of tryptophan are withdrawn from the serotonin pathway. The result is a draining, hopeless exhaustion. Some hospitals treat this problem by knocking the patient out with drugs, and feeding them whenever they wake up, before sending them straight back to sleep. Patients are often kept like this for three days.

If you don't like the idea of lying flat on your back in hospital for seventy-two hours, your body pumped full of man-made tranquillizers, try tryptophan. Tryptophan supplements restore your ability to sleep by strengthening the serotonin-producing pathway. People taking tryptophan twenty minutes before retiring find the time taken for them to get to sleep easily cut in half. Psychiatrists have discovered that it has the same antidepressant effects as drugging a patient for days on end without the harmful drug-induced side-effects. It is important that you do not take too much: Serotonin is an inhibitory neurotransmitter which is also used to treat anxiety, a highly alert mental state and virtually the opposite of depression. It is best to take no more than 250 mg ten or twenty minutes before going to bed.

High Octane Aminos

Glutamine is another excellent depression amino. As a brain fuel glutamine is essential for cell metabolism. It also helps to eliminate the toxic waste product ammonia. As the biochemist Richard Passwater says: 'The shortage of L-glutamine in the diet or glutamic acid in the brain results in brain damage due to excess ammonia or a brain that can never get into gear.' One man who was so affected by his extreme depression that he tried to kill himself was given glutamine. 'I can't believe it,' he said less than a week later. 'Is this all I have to do? I feel great. It's changed my life.'

Another turbo-boost amino is one called proline. It gives many people a sense of relief and happiness; others it actually makes angry. Either way it can elicit a positive response giving depression patients the emotional momentum they need to try to recover.

These two aminos are particularly good if you are suffering from short-term, depression. Try at least 200 mg of each, three times a day, together with 10 mg of vitamin B3 and 250 mg of vitamin C to encourage brain uptake.

Depression narrows our view of life, insisting that everything is futile, assuring us that no effort is worth making. Often, simply by giving in to these feelings they become a self-fulfilling prophecy. But they needn't be. They are, after all, only a small part of our personality but made unnaturally large by nutritional deficiencies. We all have the potential to do good, to be active in the world and, more than any form of therapy, amino acids can help us tap that potential.

Chapter 7

Anxiety Is Not All In Your Mind

Stated simply, anxiety is a stress response. Its symptoms – quickened heartbeat, the taut queasy sensation in the stomach, perspiration and heightened mental alertness – are all part of an alarm system. Your body is warning you of a stressful situation and these uncomfortable sensations are caused by its efforts to respond. This anxiety response is vital to us. It prepares us for activities that need increased physical or mental effort and even warns us away from others. It is usually short-lived. One person in twenty, though, suffers from a continual, unreasoning dread that psychiatrists call anxiety neurosis. It can inflict severe physical degeneration on victims and leave them mentally unable to face the demands of life.

What causes this extreme response? The best way to find out is by looking at a classic cause of anxiety. Then, once we understand the psychological and mental problems involved we can formulate an amino acid blend to fight it.

Red-Light Anxiety

Imagine sitting in your car at the red traffic light of a crossroad. The light changes to green. You've repeated these actions so often that you release the handbrake almost unconsciously, ease your foot off the clutch and press the accelerator. The car moves forward. Suddenly another car, running a red light, slams into your side. You are treated for shock and a few cuts and bruises, but all things considered you feel lucky to be alive.

A few weeks later you come up to the same junction. Again the light is red and the memories of the accident come vividly to life: the screech of brakes, the thundering concussion as the cars hit, tossing you sideways like a skittle, the breaking glass. Now, instead of the easy, reflexive way you usually move off, you are acutely conscious of your actions. You realize that it was exactly this chain of events that led to the accident and that every movement you now make is repeating the chain. The lights change and your throat tightens, your palm is sweaty on the gear stick and your movements are tense and jerky. The car moves off and you grit your teeth, your senses alert to danger.

The chance of being hit a second time in the same circumstances is almost non-existent. But the point is that the accident has conditioned your mind to fire the stress response whenever a similar situation arises. This sort of unrealistic fear is the source of anxiety. Our lives are full of the conditions which cause it. Perhaps as a child you were punished for sleeping in class, so that whenever you relax now you always feel guilty about it. Or you might have once been bitten by a dog leaving you terrified of them. It might even be caused by a quite unrealistic fear such as the threat of failing a job interview.

Anxiety Effects

However irrational the causes, your anxiety results from fear: of being late for work, of public-speaking or of crashing your car. When we are frightened our bodies elicit the stress response. The sympathetic nervous system fires releasing adrenalin into your body. Your heart-beat increases; your nostrils dilate; blood is diverted to the heavy muscles; and the high-frequency beta waves in your brain increase, shifting it to a state of greater alertness, watching for danger. The parasympathetic nervous system, in turn, is opposed. The low-frequency alpha waves associated with mental tranquillity diminish. Your mouth becomes dry, secretion of digestive enzymes slows down and blood is moved away from the gut. This rapid change accounts for the familiar sensations of anxiety; the rollercoaster switchback feeling in your stomach, the slight trembling and clumsiness of your muscles as they prepare for action and the acute alertness (like the person afraid of flying who notices each subtle change of pitch in the noise of the jet engine).

It leads to a sense of dread, making you feel you are about to lose something. If the anxiety continues unabated you will: your health. Without the necessary secretions of digestive acids and enzymes the food in your gut will start to putrefy and ferment. Coping with the increase in bacteria will put a stress on your immune system, leaving you more vulnerable to illness. Undigested protein seeping through into the blood will lead to allergic reactions such as fatigue, joint pains and dermatitis. The stomach lining will also suffer – ulcers are a common result of anxiety.

Most of us occasionally experience minor symptoms of anxiety – even if it's only from watching a football team we support play an important game. For some though, even the anxiety caused from this is intolerable. Their sense of dread at the outcome make it impossible for them to watch. On a wider scale the normal, everyday challenge of their lives become harder to face, forcing them to draw back from their responsibilities, and shirk confrontation.

Alleviating anxiety means having to rebalance the stress response and increase the brain's relaxing alpha waves. You can do this naturally, using specific amino acids to strengthen the inhibitory neurotransmitters in your body and encourage the parasympathetic nervous system. Or you can use Valium – and live as best you can with the side-effects as it unbalances other metabolic pathways. If you decide on the aminos there are four in particular which relieve anxiety so successfully they are often prescribed as a blend. We'll look at each in turn and see how they work.

Histidine

The first of the four is histidine – the parent molecule of the highly active amino acid histamine. One of histamine's many functions is to act as a neuro-inhibitor, reducing the intensity of beta waves in the brain and encouraging the growth of alpha wave levels. Urinary amino acid tests show that stress reduces the amount of histamine available in the cerebral cortex and hypothalamus (one of the endocrine glands responsible for the autonomic-subconscious-responses of the sympathetic and parasympathetic nervous systems). So when histamine levels are too low to control the physical and mental activity of the sympathetic (stress-reacting) nervous system, your alpha wave levels subside. The result is the sort of irritability, uncertainty and mental confusion we associate with anxiety. But by taking histidine supplements you can promote the alpha wave functions, calming and relaxing your mind when anxiety threatens to take a grip.

Histamine also helps to increase the production of gastric juices in the stomach. This offsets the digestive problems which anxiety causes, including severe indigestion and stomach ulcers. It can also relieve the allergies that may occur as the body absorbs undigested protein chains and the toxins produced by bacteria in the gut.

Sarah's case shows the importance of histidine. She is a 36-year-old computer programmer who sought help because of her anxiety. She was generally fit and followed a good nutritional programme, but she found that the high-pressure demands of her job were starting to make her irritable and confused, towards her work and her friends. Formerly proud and confident of her professionalism, she started to give way to self-doubt and an acute fear of failure. 'My ease with my work had flown out of the window,' she said, 'and I thought everyone around me was conspiring to get me sacked for my incompetence. When my manager asked me questions I was so scared about fluffing the answer that my throat constricted and all that came out were little gasps.'

A urinary analysis showed that, compared to the other amino acids in her body, her histidine levels were extremely low. A daily dose of 150 mg of histidine was prescribed and after taking it for only two weeks she reported a tremendous improvement. Her old confidence and assurance had returned and she was able to look back on her period of anxiety with amused disbelief.

Tryptophan

The second amino in our blend is tryptophan. As the precursor to the inhibitory sleep-inducing neurotransmitter serotonin, it helps to relieve anxiety simply by helping you to relax. When anxiety patients are tested their serotonin levels are usually found to be very depleted. This depletion plays a large part in making you overreact to the stimuli in life (like perspiring and gritting your teeth as you watch that ominous traffic light change from red to green). Depletion also influences the barely concealed aggression you may feel towards a person who, quite innocently, causes you to feel anxiety. And of course, if your brain doesn't have enough serotonin you simply won't be able to sleep. (see p. 59) Extra tryptophan can help to overcome all these difficulties. And, unlike the dosage for depression which has to be strictly limited, you can take it during the day.

Tryptophan is also the precursor of vitamin B3. All B vitamins are crucial for mental and emotional balance and serious deficiencies can lead to depression, schizophrenia and paranoia. A lack of B3 in particular may cause the nervousness, irritability and apprehension we associate with anxiety. As the psychlogist Abram Hoffer observed: 'If all the B3 were removed from our food everyone would be psychotic within a year.' In their book, *Psychodietetics* Drs Cheraskin and Ringsdorf tested the balancing effects of tryptophan on sixty-six volunteers. Those taking the highest doses of tryptophan (over 100 mg) described a remarkable increase in their mental composure and an almost total disappearance of anxiety.

Glycine

The third member of our alpha wave producing blend is glycine, the most commonly occurring amino in the metabolic pathways. It makes up a third of all the constituents in collagen, giving this fibrous protein the rigidity and strength it needs to structure our bodies and hold the cells together. Glycine also acts as an inhibitory neurotransmitter. Unlike histamine and tryptophan, which react in the brain, glycine works by inhibiting the nerve cells in the spinal chord. In other words, we need it to help control our motor functions – the way our bodies move. Research is showing that glycine deficiency results in jerky, exaggerated movement and sometimes even spasticity. Recently in the United States the researcher P. Stern gave glycine to seven spastic volunteers. Of these, six were delighted to find that the glycine dramatically eased their spasms and contractions, as well as improving their overall muscle tone.

How does this help your anxiety? Well, think back to your feelings as you sat in our imaginary car when the light changed to green. You know that last time, in these identical circumstances, the car crashed. The light changes and you fumble for the handbrake, pressing down so timidly on the accelerator that the car almost stalls. All these movements you usually take for granted are suddenly uncoordinated and magnified. It's as if your body isn't yours at all but a new one that you're learning to use. Now forget the car and think of the last time you personally felt extreme anxiety. You probably reacted in the same way. Although short-lived, this loss of control is similar to the effects of spasticity, which we know can be treated with glycine. Glycine works by inhibiting the messages from the spinal chord which cause these abnormal responses. Taking glycine supplements can eliminate the defective muscle control which, during anxiety, makes every movement a nightmare of self-consciousness.

Taurine

A similar rationale exists for including the fourth amino acid of the blend, taurine. Taurine is a simple sulphur-containing compound and one of the most abundant amino acids in the body. It is found in especially high concentrations in the excitable tissues such as the heart and skeletal muscle. The central nervous system also carries large amounts. Much of the research conducted into the uses of taurine centres on its function in nerve tissue and its inhibitory action on epilepsy. After an epileptic seizure the nerve tissue where the attack was centred shows very low levels of taurine. Considering the generally high concentrations elsewhere and the fact that epilepsy, like spasticity, is caused by a dysfunction of the inhibitory neurotransmitters, researchers assumed that the attacks generally occurred where levels of taurine were low. Since then it has been found highly effective in reducing seizures and is included in the formula for its powerful inhibitory action.

A well-formulated blend of free-form amino acids and co-factors should contain the following:

Aminos
tryptophan (not to be taken if you also use MAO inhibitors, see p. 192)
histidine
glycine
taurine

Co-factors
B1
B2
B6
calcium as ascorbate
C
zinc

As usual, you will need to experiment to find exactly how much suits your metabolism, taking between two and ten doses of this blend a day.

Alpha Addendums

There are two other amino acids which you might like to add to the formula. One is gamma-aminobutyric acid or GABA for short. It is important for brain metabolism and, like glycine, works in the nervous system as a neuro-inhibitor. It has been found to reduce the activity of the neurons which cause manic behaviour and acute agitation.

Finally, consider phenylalanine and tyrosine. As the precursors of the excitory neurotransmitter adrenalin you might think that this is the last amino acid you need when it comes to calming you down. In fact, these aminos have been used to great effect by many anxiety victims. Some experts think that the reason for this is that they are also the precursors of another catecholamine, L-dopa, which is used by the victims of Parkinson's disease for its neuro-inhibitory effect. It's best simply to add phenylalanine and tyrosine to the rest of the formula (unless, of course, you also take MAO inhibitors, see p. 192). If you decide to try them on their own make sure you include the important vitamin pick-ups of B6 and C.

All in all, anxiety is an unnecessary, almost superstitious fear. When you move off from that fateful crossroad you know rationally that you won't be hit again. But how do you convince your racing heartbeat, your sweaty brow and your suddenly uncoordinated limbs of the fact? Simple: whether you use them to help you stop grinding your teeth, or to relax you before an important interview, this blend of amino acids makes the gentlest, but firmest, of metabolic persuaders. Use it wisely and you may never balk at a red light again.

PART THREE

PATHWAYS TO VITALITY

Chapter 8

Master Protectors Against Illness

Earlier we compared the mass of functions and structures which make up our bodies with a city. As the inhabitants of your body-city devote themselves so selflessly to its upkeep and maintenance they are fiercely selective about who they risk allowing in to join them and what they use for building materials. To this end all-seeing, everpresent forces scrutinize every new arrival – as well as keeping a watchful eye on the natives. They are constantly alert to anything that might step out of place or pose a threat to the overall well-being. And when a danger is perceived the forces act to stamp it out, more efficiently and thoroughly than any totalitarian police state. Justice is summary and there is no appeal to a higher authority.

These brutal-sounding metabolic vigilantes are in fact the various constituents of your immune system. They guard against the constant barrage of would-be invaders – including viruses, funguses and bacteria – as well as working to slow down the ageing process caused by factors such as ultra-violet light and pollution-generated free-radicals. When one of these factors occasionally breaches the defences of your immune system and attacks the body's cells, it breaks down the complex protein structures and disrupts the metabolic pathways. The results of this invasion will range in seriousness from diarrhoea, allergies or a cold, vulnerability to debilitating viruses such as herpes and hepatitis, colitis and ulceration, to cancer and premature ageing. In future chapters we'll look at many of these problems closely and see how amino therapy, by strengthening individual metabolic pathways, can be used to fight them. And see how different blends of free-form aminos work well for different disorders.

As well as these specific formulas, we'll also recommend that you supplement your diet with a complete amino acid blend. For many people taking each free-form amino together in one supplement is every bit as important as taking them individually. Nutritionists agree that it's an invaluable nutritional aid in helping to strengthen your resistance to disease. In this chapter we'll find out why.

To save you the expense of having to buy separate containers of each amino acid then mixing them together many shops and nutritional supplement companies sell ready-mixed blends. The precise formula used may vary from company to company, but generally speaking the individual aminos are blended in the same proportions as experts have found in chickens' eggs – one of the most complete forms of protein found in nature. Many also come with the important vitamin and mineral co-factors.

You may ask why you should need to take free-form aminos separately if you are also expected to take a blend which contains them all, or, of course, why you should use a complete blend if you are taking separate aminos. The answer is that these two forms of amino therapy serve very different purposes. When you take a specific formula of two or three aminos it is to support the metabolic pathways which most directly affect your illness. But in doing so you should also keep in mind that this illness is likely to have caused a chain reaction of nutritional deficiency throughout your body – straining enzyme and hormone production, protein synthesis, the nervous system, and so on. By taking the complete blend you will help to replenish what has been lost, increasing the body's overall vitality and helping it to recover more quickly from the illness. Think of this blend as a broad, sturdy foundation which allows you successfully to build the amino therapy you need on top. Many people even include supplements of the complete blend in their daily diets to help prevent them from getting ill in the first place.

We've already looked at the individual properties of the aminos, so we know how each constituent of this complete blend will work to improve the overall well-being of your body – every one synergistically enhancing the effects of the others. Nowhere in the body is this more important than in the immune system. Put simply, every cell, every hormone and every organ of your immune system is made from protein. So taking the complete blend – even when you're not ill – provides it with the extra nutritional support to improve and strengthen its function and efficiency. Although individual aminos are used with astonishing success to relieve specific disorders, this complete blend is truly the master protector against illness.

Having the stomach for fighting

The first line of defence against literally millions of harmful, illness-causing organisms which besiege your body is the gut. Here in the stomach and intestines your body secretes the acids and enzymes which not only digest your food but also protect against fermentation, putrefaction and the build up of harmful toxins. As with the rest of the body, the gut is a fragile mechanism walking a tightrope between incredible efficiency and chronic illness. For example, the large intestine – the colon – actually contains vast numbers of bacteria such as strains of yeast with names like E.coli and lactobacilli. Harmful in themselves, they are nevertheless an important part of the digestive process. It is only the pancreas-secreted enzymes which maintain the body's uneasy relationship with these organisms. For if they were given the chance they would multiply uncontrollably, causing diseases and illness. Unfortunately, with more and more processed food being eaten this is exactly what is happening.

Fresh fruit and vegetables contain enzymes which help the body's own enzymes to prevent the food from putrefying – a state in which the bacteria flourish. Processing the food destroys many of these enzymes, and with the strain this places on the body's enzymes to meet the additional demands something has to give. It does. The bacteria population in the colon explodes and the consequences of this are numerous. For a start, with so much yeast being produced the food actually starts to ferment. The resulting alcohol is absorbed into the blood; the body reacts by lowering its blood-sugar levels and the victim begins to feel tired and run-down. At the same time the membraneous wall of the intestine starts to lose its integrity; undigested protein seep through into the bloodstream. We know that the body will only accept constituent amino acids and because of this it reacts to the presence of foreign protein with a painful allergic response – like a small-scale version of a body rejecting an organ transplant or skin graft.

There's more. The oxygen in the gut, which is needed for digestion, is consumed by some strains of the multiplying bacteria and the putrefaction to which this contributes allows dangerous toxins to escape into the bloodstream. They roam the body, replacing active neurotransmitters with inert chemicals and blocking metabolic pathways. One particularly virulent form of yeast is called candida albicans. Nutritionists in the USA are worried by the growing number of people suffering from concentrated levels of this bacteria in their colons. Evidence suggests that it can cause everything from arthritis to high blood pressure.

Think of the substances released into the body from this breakdown of proper stomach functions as the violent inmates of a maximum security prison escaping into a sleeping city and you will understand the problems your body faces. What must you do to make sure this never happens to you? Well, as the disastrous yeast growth is caused by enzyme depletion, the best way to ensure yourself against this is to raise the levels of enzymes in the gut. And you do this by taking the complete amino blend. There are at least fifteen thousand enzymes in the body with hundreds of different functions. There are cystathione synthase and glutathione synthase, which metabolize minerals in the skin and muscles; there is pepsin, an acid-tolerant enzyme secreted in the stomach, and there is a range of proteolytic-digestive enzymes such as trypsin, chymotrypsin and carboxypeptase which, as we'll see later (in Chapter 12) work to control the body's responses to food allergies. Each one is the product of metabolic pathways that occur in the pancreas from various amino acid precursors. By providing these precursors to the pancreas as part of the complete blend it can raise the levels of gut enzymes and so reduce the danger from bacteria.

The amino-derived enzymes also help to guard your body against free-radical damage. Free radicals are unstable molecules which carry an unpaired electron. In their search for an extra electron they gluttonously consume the electrons of other, balanced molecules. In doing so, they tear apart the protein structures of skin and organs causing illness and degeneration. Heavy metals and ultra-violet light cause a great deal of the free-radical destruction wrought in the body and, as antioxidants and chelators, amino acids are particularly suited to protecting the body from them. We'll see how in later chapters.

Finally, the gut also marshals large numbers of leucocytes – white blood cells – from the blood to protect the mucus lining, and these too are protein structures.

Ductless Defences

The next benefit of the complete blend for your immune system is that, as constituents of protein, amino acids are involved at every level in the function of the endocrine system. This is the group of ductless glands which include the thyroid, the gonads and the adrenal. While the frontal area of your brain controls the conscious and reasoning functions of the body, the endocrine system is controlled by the pituitary gland from an area of the brain which is much lower down the evolutionary ladder – the responses it effects are well below the conscious level. This is why it is also called the autonomic nervous system. We saw in chapter 5 how one gland – the adrenal – secretes hormones to alter the rate of the body's metabolism. That hormone, adrenalin, prepares the body for action. Another gland, the thyroid, secretes a hormone called thyroxin which is responsible for food metabolism and repair. Others include the pregnancy hormones, FSH and LH, and the pituitary-secreted growth hormone.

Another gland plays a major role in your immune response: the thymus gland. By linking a number of amino acids and co-factors, the thymus gland produces a hormone called thymosin. When this hormone is secreted it orders the spleen, together with the lymph nodes (small glands situated in various positions around your body), to manufacture T-cells, so-called because they are coded by the thymus. Imagine the T-cell response as an army, divided by the thymus into regiments of calvary, infantry and heavy artillery. Looking at each 'regiment' at a time, the cavalry are those T-cells called lymphocytes. As the army's vanguard, they circulate rapidly around the body, reconnoitring the territory, always looking out for foreign invaders. They are extremely mobile, taking advantage of the interrelationship of every part of the body with every other part. A T-cell can easily travel from a brain neuron to a cell in your little toe. It uses the main arteries and veins of the circulatory system before slipping into smaller blood vessels and finally down into the capillaries. From here it will cross into the space between blood and cell wall. Once it makes contact with the wall, the T-cell will examine it for signs of damage or infection. If the coast is clear it will leave the cell to travel elsewhere.

When lymphocytes do locate an invader they call up other regiments of their army. The first to arrive is the infantry, a group of amino-derived hormones called lymphokines. These are thought to be the body's own natural drugs and include the well-known chemical interferon. They battle with micro-organisms and toxic chemicals, breaking them down into harmless parts which the body can dispose of. If the invader is larger, the heavy artillery is brought into action – the macrophages. Literally translated, macrophage means 'big eater' and this is exactly how it works, engulfing the invader before secreting an enzyme to destroy it.

To work effectively the T-cells depend on a healthy circulatory system. Not only are blood vessels their main means of transport but the blood also supplies the thymus, spleen and lymph nodes with the nutrients they need to function. Victims of heart disorders and obesity, and heavy smokers and drinkers, often find themselves prey to minor but irritating infections. In each case their circulation is blocked by a build up of fat deposits, haemorrhaging or loss of pliability in their blood vessels. Alcohol also hardens the cells blocking the T-cell's passage. As even moderate drinking and smoking impede the immune response few of us are as healthy as we could be.

This is why the complete blend is so useful. Amino acids are the main constituents of collagen, the flexible protein structure which ensures the pliability of every blood vessel and capillary. Supplementing the body's natural resources of this protein from the complete amino blend helps to maintain its resiliency. Certain aminos from the blend, carnitine in particular, also work to mobilize and remove blockages of fat deposits; and arginine and taurine maintain the cellular membranes and improve the natural permeability of each cell. All this helps the lymphocyte to reach the area of infection much more rapidly. Furthermore, every T-cell – lymphocyte, lymphokine and macrophage – is made from amino acids with the help of vitamins (particularly vitamin C and the B complex).

The T-cell response is one branch of the body's internal defences. The other is known as the B-cell antibody, or immunoglobin, response. B-cells are made in the bone marrow from amino acid chains, and tryptophan is particularly important for this. There are five groups of antibodies and each one reacts with a different threat – one against bacteria, another against viruses, a third against toxins, and so on. They work by joining with the invading substance to render it harmless. An active and mobile germ, for example, might find itself coated with a second skin – the antibody – which serves to insulate it from any contact with the body's cells. Often when the antibody has rendered the invading substance ineffective a T-cell, such as a macrophage, will complete the process by breaking down the combined substance.

In fact, T-cells and B-cells function together in close cooperation. As well as the three T-cell regiments there are also two 'high commands' – one known as helper cells, the other called suppressors. When T-cells encounter an invading substance they produce additional helpers and these act as a signal, stimulating the production of B-cells antibodies. Suppressors, on the other hand, keep the rate of antibody production to a minimum when they are not needed. The ratio of helpers to suppressors is regulated by a substance called prostoglandin E1, which metabolizes in a four-stage metabolic pathway from a substance called linoleic acid – a chemical constituent of fatty acids. It needs amino acids to clear the pathway of any blocking agents – in particular, the action of free radicals which cause oxidation leading to rancidity of the fatty acid. We'll see in chapter 14 how this is particularly helpful when dealing with allergies – a state where, thanks to the prostoglandin-blocking agents, the immune system starts to attack itself.

The Ying and Yang of Metabolism

The next important function of the complete blend of supplements in helping protect you against illness and degeneration is that it supports the natural metabolic rhythms of your body. Every aspect of life is governed by opposing forces – action and reaction, ying and yang, work and rest, – and your body is no exception. Each day of your life it undergoes a complete anabolic/catabolic cycle. The anabolic cycle involves the processes of construction and regeneration, of manufacturing new enzymes and new protein structures. It uses up the body's existing energy. The catabolic phase is destructive. It tears down the existing protein structures, dismantles enzymes and hormones and, in doing so, releases energy.

While at first sight the anabolic phase might seem healthy and the catabolic dangerous, they are both indispensable to our vitality and well-being. Although it's true that we must be able to grow and regenerate existing tissue, it's also necessary to be able to tear old, worn-out tissue down so that the body can build anew. Before a builder can put up a new house he has to clear away the vestiges of the old, and the body is no different. In a healthy body these two phases are balanced and help to guard against illness. For instance, the growth of skin or hair is a desired, anabolic process, but the growth of a mole is also anabolic and very few people would desire this. Cancer, too, is an anabolic process and the body is usually protected from it by the tearing-down action of its catabolic phase.

An American expert in this field, Dr Emanuel Revici, conducted detailed research into this area in the early sixties, concluding that many of the illnesses which we experience result from an imbalance of this anabolic/catabolic cycle. For example, he found that viruses tend to grow when the body is in a predominantly anabolic state. Bacteria, on the other hand, as they flourish in a putrefactive – 'breaking down' – environment, do best in a catabolic body. Most illness, in fact, thrive in one cycle or the other. Revici carried his work further and found that certain food molecules are themselves anabolic and others are catabolic. Researchers have since conducted a detailed examination of a variety of nutrients to see how they affect these cycles. In the case of amino acids, while most affect the body anabolically – helping tissue build-up – one group is catabolic, assisting the body in its tearing down process.

The implications of this in terms of using it for your health are immense. As we shall see in following chapters, using amino acids to tilt the body's anabolic/catabolic balance can help you to slim, relieve heart problems, fight viruses and do much else besides. In the meantime, taking the complete amino blend will help to maintain the metabolic balance of your body, resisting virus and bacteria alike and removing the stresses from your immune system.

The advantage of the complete blend is that you can take it for many other reasons besides strengthening your immune system. If you are following a low-protein diet, for example, the complete blend will assist your body's necessary protein synthesis without raising calorie intake. It is also an excellent safeguard against possible protein deficiency if you are a vegetarian – and as free aminos are derived from plant materials they can be used by vegans. Body-builders take it with great success and some physicians are recommending it to patients awaiting, and recovering from, surgery. People suffering from digestive problems, cold intolerance, hypertension and hypotension have all benefitted from this remarkable all-inclusive blend.

Nutritionists advise a maximum of 10 grammes of the complete blend taken three times a day, for women and 15 grammes, three times a day, for men. The minimum dosage is usually around 2 grammes twice a day. One thing to make sure of when you order from a supplier or buy from a health shop is that this blend really is what the manufacturers claim it to be. The amounts of each individual amino should be printed on the side of the container. If not, it's a fair bet that the formula is overbalanced with the cheaper amino acids and you are being overcharged. By the same token don't accept hydrolized protein as an equivalent to a blend of free-form aminos. Some manufacturers will take a protein powder, sprinkle in a negligible quantity of amino acids, then prominently display the fact that they are included, giving a distorted impression of what you are buying; for all it really is, is an expensive protein which the body has to digest. If you are taking the blend to improve your digestion, for example, this is not what you want. In other words, make sure that you are getting the right product at a fair price.

Chapter 9

Sex and Amino Acids

Sexual problems, in one form or another, are widespread and can be a source of intense suffering and anxiety. Frigidity, sterility and impotence are not only unpleasant in themselves; they are also major causes of stress.

The sex drive in all animals, including man, is one of the deepest biological urges. In man, sex also plays a major role in developing deeper emotional relationships. Through the simultaneous act of possession and surrender, in this most consuming of actions, we achieve a physical and emotional intimacy inexpressible in any other way.

When sex works for us it can make us feel rich emotionally and physically. It also brings us closer to our partners and makes us more loving. Unfortunately, it doesn't work for everyone. For those who have experienced frigidity, impotence and other difficulties sex can become a mixture of frustration, anger and resentment – bringing them a sense of unjust imprisonment in a body that confounds passion. Fulfilment depends not only upon emotional factors. For sex to work things have to be right biochemically. This is where amino acids can be helpful. For by strengthening the relevant metabolic pathways it is possible to banish impotence, cure frigidity and even stimulate fertility, providing real hopes of childbirth for many childless couples.

In Search of Orgasm

Perhaps the most widespread sexual problem today is the difficulty many women have in achieving orgasm. Until now, non-orgasmic women have been given psychotherapy, often without results. Even the unkind, almost rebuking term which describes this condition, 'frigidity', suggests a mental attitude in the sufferer – an offhandedness or lack of passion – rather than a physical inability. Recently, however, research has shown that frigidity is often physiological in origin. It can be corrected by supplementing the diet with a combination of specific free-form amino acids such as lysine, arginine and histidine. Of these, the most important free-form amino is histidine.

Histidine needs to be present in good quantity for orgasm to take place. This amino acid is the parent of the active molecule histamine. Orgasm is triggered when histamine is released in the body from the mast cells in the genitals. These cells, which are present in all organic matter, especially the soft tissues of the body, function as part of the immune system. In fact, the body's response to infection – reddening, watering and swelling – is caused by histamine release in the affected cells. The link between this response and the sexual flush experienced during arousal has been recognized for years. And the active ingredient in both reactions is histamine. Scientists have recently discovered that when there is insufficient histidine in the body, histamine production is low and women find it difficult, sometimes even impossible, to achieve orgasm. The result is frigidity with its destructive by-products of guilt and anger.

The effects on orgasm of histamine have been well documented for over a decade by the American researcher Carl Pfeiffer. Yet old notions die hard. The standard treatment for so-called frigid women is still some kind of psychotherapy. To counter this view, Pfeiffer conducted a study on frigid women. He discovered that, in addition to their frigidity, many of the women he tested were also victims of extreme fatigue and anxiety. Others had only experienced orgasm during the early stages of adolescence and subsequently lost interest altogether. Pfeiffer was not surprised to find, therefore, that most of his subjects suffered from low levels of many of the amino acids. But their histamine levels were particularly low. He reasoned that by giving these women extra histidine they might experience orgasm for the first time. It worked. Without any psychotherapy the bodies of the women who had been given histidine broke the bonds of frigidity, bringing an enormous sense of liberation in its wake. Since then histidine has often been used in this way by a number of sophisticated nutritional counsellors. It is either given in the form of a 500 mg dose before each meal or as part of a larger and better balanced sex formula, which we will look at more closely at the end of the chapter.

Pfeiffer also says that 4 grammes or more of histidine can bring on an early menstrual period. In fact, some women have actually used histidine to time their cycles in this way and so prevent the pain and inconvenience interfering at awkward times – such as at a wedding or an athletics meeting.

Too much too soon

Pfeiffer also examined the benefit of histidine for men, discovering what a two-edged sword it is. Male orgasm is a localized reflex caused by the release of histamine from a large concentration of mast cells in the penis head. As expected, the circulating levels of histidine played a significant role, both in the ability of a man to climax and in the time it takes him. The higher the levels, the shorter the time needed – so much so that for a few this led to another problem: premature ejaculation.

Premature ejaculation can bring to a man many of the same feelings of frustration, shame and embarrassment that frigidity can to a woman. What is more it is usually diagnosed in the same catch-all manner as a 'psychological' problem. Supplementing a patient's histidine levels to cure frigidity is one thing, but finding a way of lowering those levels is quite another. The discovery of how it could be done came as a result of work with the mentally disturbed. Pfeiffer found that many schizophrenics have inordinately high levels of histidine. He also discovered that if he gave them supplements of the amino acid methionine it would rebalance things.

Then he extended his studies to men suffering from premature ejaculation as a result of their own high histamine levels. He discovered that these too could be lowered by methionine given with a little calcium as a co-factor. These men are now able to lead more satisfying sex lives. How does it all work? Rather than directly competing with histidine, the methionine is converted by the action of a magnesium-dependent enzyme into its active form s-adenosyl methionine – the substance which, as we saw in chapter 2, is needed to create adrenalin. And as we'll see in a moment, adrenalin is a most important chemical in controlling the body's sexual activity. In this case it works by mitigating the effects of high histamine levels and so delays orgasm. Unfortunately, as methionine is a sulphur-based amino it has an unpleasant rotten egg odour – something which many men all too willingly put up with to be free of premature ejaculation. The odour needn't be a problem at all if you opt for 500 mg capsules or tablets instead of the powder. In helping people deal with premature ejaculation, most nutritionists suggest they take 1500 mg of methionine – together with 300–500 mg of magnesium and 50 mg of vitamin B6 as co-factors – divided into three daily doses.

Amino Keys to Fertility

But good sex is not always an end in itself. At some point most people want children. Yet many have their hopes tragically unfulfilled. With the expanding world population, some cultures, faced with the demands placed on their limited agricultural and economic resources, are starting to regard childbirth as an unaffordable luxury. In China, for example, the authorities are checking their massive population build-up by allowing only one child for each couple – a terrible irony for couples in the West physically unable to conceive at all. For all of them it is a disappointing and frustrating time. For a few – those who see having children as the *raison d'etre* of their relationship – it can even threaten a breakdown. Even in the most balanced and open of relationships infertility can create enormous strains.

A major cause of this problem lies in low sperm count. In recent years the average sperm count of men in the West has decreased dramatically. No one knows why. Some scientists attribute it to the cumulative polluting and poisoning of the planet. Others see the additives we use to process our foods, or the hormones fed to livestock as responsible. Whatever the cause, the fact is that the average male sperm count has declined from 100 million per cubic centimetre at the turn of the century to less than 25 million today – dangerously close to the level of sterility. Too many men have now fallen beneath it.

Amino acids can come to the rescue here as well. As long ago as 1926 research into the composition of semen revealed the presence of the two amino acids which we now call spermadine and spermine. But it wasn't until the mid-1960s that they were found to play a major role in the synthesis of semen. It is these two amino acids which give semen its characteristic odour. More important, tests carried out on vasectomy patients and women using the contraceptive pill (two groups which, like men suffering from low sperm count, have undergone a loss of fertility) showed much lower concentrations of the two amino acids than people outside these groups. It was therefore logical for biochemists to assume that supplements of the amino acid parent molecule of spermadine and spermine, given to men suffering from low sperm count, would ease their problems. And indeed it has.

The parent amino acid in this metabolic pathway is arginine. Through the action of manganese, vitamin B6 and most especially methionine (whose influence on histamine we have already seen), arginine undergoes a conversion process first to ornithine, then to putrescine, spermadine and finally spermine (see p. 41). Again we see a complex co-relationship of factors needed to bring about the smooth running of the metabolic pathways: arginine may be the single most important element of this pathway but the presence of helpers such as methionine is essential.

In one recent study forty-two men suffering from low sperm count were given arginine together with its co-factors. Each patient showed an almost 100 per cent increase in his sperm count shortly after the trials began. Better still, the motility – the ability of the individual sperm to move – was also greatly increased. This is important if the sperm is to reach the egg so that ovulation can occur. When researchers withdrew the arginine the sperm count immediately dropped. It rose again when the amino acid was readministered.

The maximum recommended dose of arginine for the treatment of low sperm count is 8 grammes a day. Like all the amino acids used to improve metabolic pathways it relies on certain co-factors. These include vitamins B6, B1, B2, C and some other amino acids. The sex formula at the end of this chapter is an excellent way of getting them all.

To Have and to Hold

Even after successfully raising the male sperm count, his partner might still be unable to conceive, often because of undetected nutritional deficiencies. If this is the case amino acid supplements can also greatly increase her chances.

A successful pregnancy needs the support of two important hormones: follicle-stimulating hormone (FSH) which is mainly responsible for the growth and development of the ovaries, and leutenizing hormone (LH) whose chief function is to promote ovulation. The composition of both these hormones include long chains of amino acids. Of course, a full and balanced supply of all the essential amino acids is vital in the formation of the hormone molecules. The cysteine content in these two hormones is particularly high, so this amino is especially important. FSH production can be diminished by the inhibiting effects of the neurotransmitter hormone serotonin. Since the amino acid tryptophan is the parent molecule of serotonin it can be reduced by the action on tryptophan of a competing amino acid such as phenylalanine or tyrosine. As well as these amino acids, Vitamin C helps the replenishment of the ovaries (especially when their growth is being stimulated by the action of FSH) and vitamin E is important for the maintenance of the cell membrane of the sex organs. A nutritional programme for infertility needs to be carefully tailored to a couple's individual needs. However, most are based around a daily balance of nutrients which looks something like this:

Aminos

arginine	in two doses
cysteine	in two doses
histidine	in three doses
methionine	in two doses
phenylalanine	in two doses

Co-factors

B3	at each meal
B6	at each meal
E	at each meal
folic acid	at each meal
zinc citrate	once a day
selenium methionate	once a day
magnesium aspartate	once a day

Post Natal Help

Even after conceiving, some women find themselves faced with the threat of a miscarriage. The most important hormone during pregnancy is progesterone and, to put it simply, if progesterone is deficient the pregnancy will end prematurely. On the other hand, if you have too much progesterone, pregnancy will be extended beyond its natural span. Unlike FHS and LH, progesterone is not an amino acid structure. The most important molecule in this pathway is cholesterol. Pregnant women musn't try to avoid it in their diets. In this area, too, metabolic nutrition based on free-form amino acids can be enormously helpful. A daily formula for helping to maintain pregnancy might look something like this:

Aminos
glutamine
tryrosine
lysine
proline
leucine
isoleucine
valine

Co-factors

B1
B2
B6
B12
C
E
folic acid
niacin
zinc

Sex and stress

We've looked at specific sexual problems and conditions and at the amino acids which can help remedy them. Sexual ability, however, also depends upon the body's general state of wellbeing. Here too amino acids play a prominent role – particularly thanks to the aminos phenylalanine and tyrosine. Tyrosine, combines with the mineral iodine in the thryroid gland to produce thyroxin – a hormone which controls your body's rate of cellular metabolism. Without sufficient thyroxin the body becomes lethargic and sluggish. Then decision-making is difficult without that 'first cup of coffee'; you are easy prey to stress. There is also a loss of interest in physical activity – including sex. Making sure your thyroid gland has enough tyrosine to produce thyroxin is vital in ensuring good health, and specifically, sexual activity.

Tyrosine is created from its parent amino acid, phenylalanine, by the relatively simple action of the enzyme phenylalanine carboxy-lase with a substance derived from folic acid. Phenylalanine also supports sexual activity through a complicated metabolic pathway which affects the production of adrenalin.

Sexual performance is maintained by a complex interaction of two branches of the autonomic nervous system. While one branch, the sympathetic, is responsible for the fight-or-flight stress response, the other, the parasympathetic, is responsible for the body-at-rest functions such as digestion. The two actually relate synergistically: it is the balance between the two systems that ensures adequate responses in a given situation. For example, even though the sympathetic nervous system prepares your body for the stress situation of sex by secreting adrenalin (which raises blood pressure and increases circulation to the lungs and muscles), if the stress becomes too great (perhaps because of extreme nervousness) the body will simply be unable to perform. Such are the acrobatic complexities of balancing the parasympathetic with the sympathetic branch of the autonomic nervous system. To maintain this balance, responding evenly to the stress demands that sex makes on the body, a healthy circulating level of adrenalin, determined to a great extent by the action phenylalanine, is vital.

Carnitine – the Don Juan Amino

Another amino acid whose presence affects sexual performance is L-carnitine. It is made from the amino acids lysine and methionine and is used in the treatment of ischemic heart disease (where insufficient oxygen reaches the heart, reducing its ability to pump blood around the body). Basically, carnitine is needed to transport fatty acids into and out of the cellular membranes. Therefore, it plays a key role in ensuring that muscles are supplied with the energy that they need to respond even to most extreme demands of love-making. Used for this purpose carnitine is given in doses of between 1000 and 1500 mg a day. It is best taken together with the following complete sex formula.

This formula consists of combinations of free-form aminos with their vitamin and mineral hook-ups – substances known to offer the best help which until the advent of metabolic nutrition was simply unavailable. The nutrients should be taken in split doses throughout the day.

Aminos
histidine
arginine
lysine
methionine
phenylalanine
tyrosine

Co-factors
B1
B2
B6
C
pantothenic acid
folic acid
niacin
copper
magnesium aspartate

selenium methionate
zinc citrate
manganese

Overall high-level health is of immense importance in making sex work for you. Amino acids are basic to good health, contributing to all enzyme systems, cellular repair, hormone production, and so on. In truth, our bodies are so finely balanced that the metabolic equilibrium is easily disrupted. When this happens the body's functions begin to break down. Sexual disability is often a result of this fine metabolic disruption. To those who feel they are living in a prison of anxiety, bitterness and bewilderment over sex the right amino acids can be the long-sought key to freedom.

Chapter 10

Digestive Trouble – A Thing of the Past

Digestion is a crucial part of the body's metabolic equation. It is the balance between the food you eat and the use your body makes of it. Suffering from poor digestion upsets this balance and causes your body more harm than you probably imagine. You may eat an excellent diet with a full balance of all the vitamins, minerals and proteins you need. But if the food isn't digested properly your body simply won't be able to grow and repair as it should.

We've all suffered from an 'upset' or 'acid' stomach. Most of us have probably embarrassed ourselves in company with an accidental burp or 'wind'. Usually these things are only symptoms of a mildly unsettled gut. Occasionally, though, they may signify that something is giving your digestion serious trouble. If you smoke, for example the chances are high that you suffer from depleted stomach acids and enzyme levels. Constipation and/or gut-dumping often result from allergies you might have. The stress of emotional difficulties can lead to ulcers and colitis. Even the quality of the food itself is often to blame for your problems.

Whatever the cause, the simple fact is that when your digestion doesn't work as it should your cells are starved of the nutrients they need for healthy living. Toxins are allowed to build up which cause oxidation and cell degeneration. Growth and resistance to disease is reduced. Your skin gets blotchy; your body feels heavier and more sluggish; and your emotions become exaggerated and unstable. Remember, your digestive system is a pipeline carrying vitality from the food to your cells. Bad digestion cuts that pipeline off.

Amino acids could have been invented for these problems. In their free-form state, separated from the long protein molecule chains, the gut isn't needed to break them down. For all intents and purposes they are 'pre-digested'. They pass quickly and easily through the gut wall into the bloodstream. And from there they can help to reestablish normal digestive functions, strengthening the pancreas and stimulating the production of digestive acids and enzymes. In this chapter we'll follow your food on its passage through the gut. Then, seeing where and how problems arise, we can prescribe amino formulas which will help to restore the delicate digestive balance between your food and your body.

Acid Remarks

In the food-rich West we overeat. The opportunities for over-indulgence, not to say gluttony, are everywhere: on holidays, at parties, in restaurants and on the overflowing shelves of super-markets. The problem with this abundance is that many people simply do not have enough stomach acid to cope with it. In their book *Psychodietetics* Drs Cheraskin and Ringsdorf record their examination of over three thousand victims of gastrointestinal disorders. They found that the problems of a third of this group stemmed simply from insufficient stomach acid.

Stomach acid is important because it is the first stage of digestion. Any problems here will be magnified enormously by the time the food passes into your intestines. Let's see why.

Usually, when it reaches the stomach, your food activates the release of hydrochloric acid. This acid environment is important for stimulating the enzyme pepsin into action. Pepsin digests approxi-mately 15 per cent of the food before it passes on to the small intestine. But for those people who suffer from low stomach acid – caused perhaps by smoking, heavy drinking or even as part of the natural process of ageing – the percentage will be much less. One of the first results of this drop in stomach acid is that the food will literally start to ferment. Here's why: as well as its own acids and enzymes, your body permits the growth of a certain amount of bacteria and yeast to aid digestion. As we discovered in chapter 8, the threat of any dangerous expansion of the gut's yeast colony is kept in check by the acids and enzymes. We also saw how stresses inhibit enzyme production and allow the yeast to flourish. Insufficient acid, leading to low pepsin levels, is one such stress. It lets the yeast colony become so metabolically overactive that it causes fermenta-tion. Large quantities of carbohydrate are turned into alcohol. This is the same process that has been used throughout history to make spirits; your gut, in effect, becomes a still. In some cases this is so serious that victims literally get drunk on the carbohydrate they eat. It distorts consciousness, puts massive stresses on their liver and kidneys and often leads to obesity and hypoglycemia. Like ordinary alcoholics needing a drink, they simply cannot live without eating increasing amounts of carbohydrate food.

Few people realize that this can be traced back to a yeast problem in the gut – still fewer that low stomach acid levels are directly responsible. We estimate that as many as nine out of ten stomach upsets mistakenly attributed to acid indigestion – too much acid in the gut – are actually the result of yeast fermentation from too little acid. The common response? Reach for the antacid tablets, of course. As this only serves to reduce acid levels still further it is the worst thing you can do.

But the consequences of low stomach acid don't end here. Worse is to come as the undigested, fermenting food, reaches the small intestine. This is where the pancreas usually secretes digestive enzymes – a different one for each amino acid link of the protein chain – together with a buffering solution to regulate what acid is brought with the food from the stomach, in an ideal body at least. But with your body already under the stresses caused by depleted stomach acid, the pancreas can't cope with the increased quantity of undigested food. Much of the food, therefore, just sits in the gut and putrefies like a rubbish tip and this decomposition releases potentially harmful substances. For example, instead of liberating phenylalanine – precursor of the catecholamine neurotransmitters – the bacterial activity converts it to phenylethylamine (PEA). Unable to distinguish between the two, the gut wall absorbs it just the same. When PEA reaches the brain it is transformed into the pseudo-neurotransmitter octopamine, replacing the active neuro-transmitter noradrenalin. The results of this may range from subtle changes of behaviour – how well you remember and think – to severe emotional problems like anxiety, depression and even schizophrenia.

With this runaway putrefaction, histamine, too, is released from your food instead of its precursor, histidine. Elsewhere in the body histamine is active in the body's immune response, sexual functions and neuro-inhibitory activity. In the small intestine, however, it causes an allergic reaction and forces the intestine wall to secrete mucinous substances to protect itself. In time this leads to diarrhoea and gut-dumping. Putrid smelling flatulence and faeces and a powerful, unpleasant body odour are common physical symptoms of putrefaction.

Remember, all the problems we've looked at so far stem from depleted stomach acid. And the implications of this depletion go beyond even these serious health problems. Look at this quote from Newbold's *Vitamin C Against Cancer*: 'I have found... that (cancer) patients are either hypo- or achlohydric (little or no stomach acid). In order for them to get any nutrition you've got to supplement their stomach acid.'

The first thing to do then is to raise the stomach acid levels in your gut to allow digestion to take place. Free-form 'pre-digested' amino acids are excellent for this. They will be absorbed by the body, even though the acid and enzyme levels are low. Furthermore, many experts believe that because individual free-form aminos are not complete foods in themselves, they won't be attacked by the ravenous bacterial population. So which are the most helpful?

First, we recommend a supplement containing the complete amino blend. As almost every enzyme depends on amino acids for its structure, when digestion is inefficient your body is robbed of the nutrients it needs to create these enzymes. To combat this problem some people take the enzymes themselves as supplements. But before these supplements can begin to act on the food they first have to run the gauntlet of the digestive process and often they are broken down in the stomach before doing any good. The complete amino blend is a much more reliable alternative to enzyme supple-mentation. It contains the nutrients the body needs to manufacture its enzymes from scratch. This blend – the 'master protector against illness' – also helps to rid the body of many of the ill effects of poor digestion. As a group, amino acids provide nutritional 'first aid' to depleted cells. Aminos like carnitine and glutathionine clear blood vessels of toxins and fats. And phenylalanine, tyrosine and methionine help to improve your emotional stability and mental alertness, replacing the imposter neurotransmitters with the potent catecholamines.

Specifically to help raise your acid levels your diet should include additional amounts of glutamic acid HCL, tryptophan, histidine and glycine. Glutamic acid HCL is a widely available free-form amino supplement mixed with hydrochloric acid. Providing hydrochloric acid like this is the quickest and most direct way of raising the stomach acid levels to help digestion. Glutamic acid itself has several important digestive functions. In the case of people with high carbohydrate intake and gut fermentation it helps to regulate blood sugar levels. This eases the stress on the insulin-producing pancreas, allowing it instead to secrete the necessary proteolytic enzymes into the small intestine.

Glutamine, the amine form of glutamic acid, has been found to help decrease alcohol consumption by working on the appetite centres in the hypothalamus. In this way, your carbohydrate-dependency can be reduced, in turn cutting down the degree of carbohydrate fermentation in the stomach and small intestine. Glutamine is produced by the action of glutamic acid on the toxic ammonia in the brain. The destructive action of ammonia on the brain cells causes a variety of mood-associated disorders. As these may in turn lead to gastrointestinal problems the ammonia-flushing action of glutamic acid is important.

Many people also get tremendous help from tryptophan. If we follow the metabolic pathway from tryptophan towards the production of niacin (B3) we come across a substance called nicotinamide-adenine-dinucleotide (NAO). As well as playing an important role in alleviating mood disorders NAO also helps to stimulate the production of stomach acid.

What about the two remaining digestion-helping aminos on our list, histidine and glycine? In the stomach – as opposed to the intestines – histamine (the amine form of histidine) promotes natural stomach acid secretion. It also increases the amount of saliva in the mouth. Glycine, too, by converting to the digestive chemical, betaine, improves acid secretion. In fact, nutritionists are now prescribing betaine as a supplement itself, together with HCL. Here's an acid-stimulating formula you might try:

Aminos
glutamic acid HCL
tryptophan (not to be taken by people on MAO inhibitors see p. 192)
histidine
glycine
betaine HCL

Co-factors
B3
B6
C as ascorbic acid

The value of these amino acid supplements simply cannot be overstated. A good analogy is to examine the sprinter's starting blocks at an athletics meeting. In a race, where the margin of victory is measured in hundredths of a second, the blocks must be set perfectly to give a sprinter the maximum possible impetus as he pushes off. If they are wrongly spaced or, if he starts without any blocks at all, he might be the fastest man alive, but in his efforts to catch up with the other competitors he will overstride, lose his natural rhythm and come last. Stomach acid is your digestive starting block. As the food you eat is only as good as the way it is digested, this amino acid formula will give it precisely the start it needs.

More Problems Further Down

You would be wrong to think that all your problems stem from low stomach acid and enzyme levels. An increasingly common problem in our refined food age is the lack of fibre in our diets. Fibre is the undigestible part of the food which helps the muscle contractions of the gut wall – peristalsis – to draw it through the alimentary canal. The time it takes normal, high fibre food to pass through the body is between twenty-four and forty-eight hours. The less fibre you have in your diet, though, the longer it will take. Many people suffer from transit times of four days or more.

This is itself a cause of serious intestinal disorders. First, as it moves so slowly the faeces lose water through the gut wall, becoming harder and more rasping in the process. The greater physical friction of the passing food with the gut causes small pouches to form on the intestine wall. These pouches – called diverticulosis – only serve to slow the food even further. The longer the food remains in the gut, the more damage the toxic by-products will do. Nitrosamine compounds, for example – a mixture of bile salt secretions and nitrates – can cause anything from varicose veins, to appendicitis and even cancer of the colon. Also, undigested protein starts to leak through the gut wall, causing allergic reactions. If you often feel bloated and sluggish, even a long time after eating, excrete very hard stools and suffer from headaches and unaccountable joint pains this could be your problem.

But these physical symptoms aren't all. In the large intestine the diverticulosis pouches often become inflamed: this is called diverticulitis. It can lead to the discomfort and suffering of ulcers, rectal bleeding and haemorrhoids. But, in addition to the physical pain, many psychologists now recognize a connection between this and severe mental disturbances. Accumulating in the pouches, often over many years, the bacteria and toxic by-products may be responsible for abnormal anxiety, tension, manic depression, and perhaps even schizophrenia. It is almost unheard of for colitis sufferers to be unaffected by these problems. Traditionally, doctors believed that stress could affect intestinal disorders – by slowing down digestive functions – but not vice versa. It now seems probably that intestinal problems are just as likely to cause stress. Each effectively helps perpetuate the other.

Recognizing the link between the two, many experts find that one of the best forms of treatment is the amino anxiety formula – tryptophan, histidine, taurine and glycine – taken at least an hour before a high fibre meal together with phenylalanine. The fact that tryptophan and histidine are already included in this chapter to help raise stomach acid levels shows the remarkable multi-purpose qualities of amino acids. In this case they perform quite different functions.

Both tryptophan and histidine are powerful neuro-inhibitors. High histamine levels in the hypothalamus increase the calming alpha wave activity of your brain. These brain waves help your body's parasympathetic nervous system to operate effectively. This is the side of your autonomic nervous system that is responsible for digestive functions – for pumping blood to the gut and stimulating peristalsis. Additional histidine, therefore, helps the gut to digest your food more efficiently. Tryptophan, as the precursor of serotonin, also soothes your mental activity. So when stress does occur it lets your body cope with it a lot more effectively. This ensures that blood needed for digestion will stay in the gut rather than being diverted to the heavy muscles as part of the stress response. It also allows enzyme secretion to continue as normal.

Unlike histidine and tryptophan, which work in the brain, glycine and taurine inhibit the excitory actions of the central nervous system. This has the effect of relaxing the bowel muscles, allowing smoother peristaltic contractions and quicker transit times.

Taken before your high fibre meal the anxiety formula is invaluable in helping your body to get the full nutritional benefit from its food. Then, once digested, it ensures that the waste products will be ejected smoothly and quickly, preventing a harmful build up of toxins.

Philip is a mountaineer in his late thirties, leading an active and vigorous life in Scotland. 'I've always been very moody,' he said, 'I used to like putting it down to a "volatile Celtic temperament". The trouble was that last year I went from the occasionally irritable to the downright unstable. I started going through fits of bottomless, black depression. Any mental effort seemed to be too much. I remember once bursting into tears when I couldn't think of a word I wanted to use in an article I was writing. At the same time my body lost its vitality. I could hardly walk upstairs without my legs feeling like lead, let alone walk up a mountain.' His dismay deepened when he noticed that varicose veins had appeared on his calves. Furthermore, during this period – about eight months – he gained nearly a stone in weight.

Describing these and other symptoms – stiff joints, a craving for sweets and cakes and painfully hard stools – it was clear that Philip was suffering from chronic digestive difficulties. He was prescribed the complete amino digestive programme: the anxiety formula (p.

66), together with phenylalanine, beltaine HCL and glutamic acid to satisfy his carbohydrate craving – all supplementing a diet high in fibre.

Within three weeks his body felt clearer – mentally and physically – than it ever had in his life. 'I realized all that stuff about the dour Celtic moodiness was rubbish,' he admitted. 'It was as if I'd been perceiving my life through a dirty windscreen. Now that it's clean I can't believe how I ever managed before. As for my body it feels lighter, more resilient and I have to walk twice as far to burn up all the energy.'

Down and Out

As well as amino acids, fibre was important in helping Philip to recover. A few words of warning, though: when you decide on the high-fibre diet to accompany the amino formulas, beware of the pitfalls. Many people mistakenly think that bran will satisfy all their fibre needs. In fact, bran is quite harmful. Its scraping action often irritates an already inflamed bowel. When this happens the gut wall secretes mucus to protect itself. This has the effect of making the food pass rapidly through the body to give the bowel a chance to heal itself. If the bemused victim of constipation suddenly finds himself suffering from diarrhoea this could be the cause. Bran also raises your sugar levels and decreases the absorption of important minerals like magnesium and zinc. Instead of bran why not try increasing your consumption of other natural fibre sources such as grains, and fresh fruit and vegetables? Their colon-cleansing action is far better than bran. After all, which would you use on your car, a chamois cloth or a brillo pad? These non-irritating bran sources will also help to regulate your blood sugar levels.

The Gut Dumpers

For most people diarrhoea is unpleasant but short-lived. Some however, as a result of an allergy perhaps or an irritated bowel, suffer chronically. It is a deceptively dangerous problem as it prevents the victim from getting any benefit from their food at all. The gut wall simply has no time to absorb the nutrients. This is known as gut dumping and if it is allowed to continue it can lead to severe malnourishment. Sufferers are often thin, finding it impossible to put on any weight however much they eat. In the cases of young children it can be particularly serious as it might halt their growth altogether. Happily, gut dumping responds particularly well to high doses of the complete amino blend. In the early stages of recovery the victim's gut is often so sensitive that amino acids and their co-factors – having no bulk or fibre – are the only things it will tolerate.

Chapter 11

Help Against Herpes

'What's the difference between love and herpes?' 'Simple. Herpes last forever.' This joke is as old as the current herpes epidemic. It neatly sums up the reason for the sudden despair and isolation felt by many victims when they contract the virus. Quite simply, herpes is unlike any other sexual problem. While couples who suffer from the heartache of impotence or frigidity can, after all, still share a physical intimacy – still sleep together regardless of their problems – herpes is different. This highly infectious, excrutiatingly painful virus brands victims with the physical stigma of lesions and cold sores. It renders the reassuring intimacy with a lover almost impossible without the threat of passing on the infection, regardless of precautions. And there is no known cure.

With their ability to strengthen the body's natural defences, however, amino acids represent perhaps the most potent form of herpes prevention known. Even if you are unlucky enough to have contracted the virus already there are amino acid formulas which are providing relief to thousands of victims. Let's see how herpes attacks the body. Then, by pinpointing the areas which it affects, we can formulate a metabolic programme which will help to ease a sufferer's sense of isolation and agony.

There are two forms of herpes infection: simplex-one which affects the mouth with large scrabrous sores and blisters, and simplex-two which affects the genitals in much the same way but with often intense pain. The herpes virus lives in the nerve cells. By attaching itself to the cell wall, it injects the cell with its own DNA. As DNA determines the characteristics of living things, this has the effect of adapting the nerve cell to obey the commands of the virus. This allows it to multiply. It spreads down the nerves to the skin, causing the highly infectious lesions to erupt on the surface. Each outbreak may last for anything from a week to several months. Even when the lesions disappear the virus is still present in the nervous system. It lies dormant, waiting until the metabolic conditions are ripe for it to spread again. Knowing what these metabolic conditions are, and why they allow the virus to prosper, is crucial in helping to decide which supplements to use.

Stress and herpes

Doctors are finding that people regularly contract herpes, and that symptoms recur in existing victims, following periods of stress. This is because the metabolic imbalances that stress causes deplete their bodies of the nutrients which provide them with their natural immunity. Without a vigorous immune system to repel it the virus can develop much more freely. Furthermore, finding you have contracted herpes is a highly stressful discovery in itself. The anxiety it causes can only lead to greater nutritional deficiencies. 'I couldn't believe I'd caught it,' said one victim, 'I couldn't eat. I couldn't sleep. I was so worried. I thought: "This is it. This is the end." I was absolutely panic-stricken.'

This attitude almost guarantees regular recurrences of the virus. For the last thing you can afford to do when you contract herpes is to squander your body's valuable metabolic resources by giving in to stress and anxiety. Uncontrolled stress is like a runaway train, relentlessly gathering speed and momentum: when the train finally hits the buffers at the end of the line the impact is enormous. The same thing happens to a stressed body when it 'runs into' an infection.

What you must try to do instead of simply worrying is to make sure that your body is equipped nutritionally to withstand the stress. We've already seen how disastrous the results of a poor diet – and the digestive disorders it causes – are in terms of resisting stress and strengthening your immune system to fight infection. The knock-on effect that each metabolic imbalance causes elsewhere in the body seriously undermines your health and vitality. So when the herpes virus attacks, your immune system is simply too tired to resist it.

Physical Resistance

With amino acid supplements we can protect our bodies from the physical and mental ravages of stress. This will leave us much more resistant to attacks from the herpes virus. So which nutrients should we choose to give us the best protection? This formula may prove useful when taken three times a day between meals:

Aminos
tyrosine*
DL-phenylalanine*
glutamic acid

methionine
*do not take if you are using MAO inhibitors (see p. 192)

Co-factors
B3
B6
C
magnesium aspartate

What does this formula do? Going through each substance in turn, glutamic acid combines in the brain with the harmful waste-product ammonia to produce the brain fuel glutamine. By clearing away this toxicity – which builds up so quickly during stress – it will leave you much more alert and composed. As a brain fuel, glutamine will help to alleviate the torpor and aparthy of depression. This is crucial when you need all your energy and determination to fight the infection.

DL-phenylalanine is the precursor of tyrosine and the cate-cholamines noradrenalin and adrenalin. Like glutamine, nor-adrenalin is an antidepressant which almost literally 'charges' your brain. Adrenalin is the driving force of the stress response. More than simply furnishing you with the energy to respond to stress, it helps to contain any overreaction such as anxiety. In this way it plugs the drain of vital nutrients which happens so easily during stress.

DL-phenylalanine is also a proven painkiller. By preventing the brain enzyme enkephalinase from breaking down the body's natural opiates, it can give substantial relief against the pain of the herpes lesions. As pain itself is a major stressor, you can see that the help that DLPA gives is vital. Methionine is included in the formula because it is necessary for the conversion of noradrenalin to adrenalin.

Mental Resistance

This amino-based stress formula is one of the best nutritional support programmes you can give your body. But it will be even more effective in strengthening your resistance to infection if you can raise your stress threshhold. Experts now realize the importance of conditioning yourself to withstand stress – without your sympathetic nervous system firing. If, for example, you can sit in a traffic jam for hours, or be woken up at three in the morning by street-revellers, without feeling anxiety or anger, then fewer essential nutrients will need to be diverted away from your immune system.

There are several methods of raising your stress threshold which nutritionists are successfully using in conjunction with amino acid therapy. One very popular method is biofeedback. This is simply a method of learning to control the bodily processes which occur involuntarily, using the 'feedback' of sensitive measuring instruments to guide you. For example, let's say you want to ease a migraine caused by stress. You might decide to attach a sensor to your hand which measures skin temperature. You would then try to imagine that the sun is shining on it – concentrating acutely on the feel of its imaginary warmth covering your skin. When the sensation becomes vivid the capillaries in your hand will dilate. This happens because your body has been fooled into thinking that one small area is hotter than the rest. As it wants to maintain an even temperature it will pump blood to the skin surface to release heat. This in turn will lower the blood pressure in other parts of your body including your forehead and so relieve the migraine.

The biofeedback instrument itself provides no relief but, by showing the rise in skin temperature, acts as a guide in helping you to develop your imaginative skill. With practice, you will find that you won't even need the equipment allowing you to ease your stress symptoms almost at will.

Another simple and effective method of stress control is meditation. According to The Friends of the Healing Research Trust, 'meditation frees the mind from its enslavement to discursive thoughts with their attendant feelings which together dissipate energy and cause stress and suffering.' Putting aside fifteen or twenty minutes a day you can practise it at home. Sit quietly in a chair with your feet on the floor. Close your eyes, breathe deeply and relax. Choose a simple word like 'one'. Then, blocking out everything else – all your anxieties – repeat it continuously to yourself. If you become distracted or feel your mind wandering, gently guide it back to the word and carry on repeating it.

Alpha Aid

Concentrating wholly on this word will seem impossible at first. Your mind will disobediently race from one preoccupation to another. If this happens don't give up. Many patients who find they are easily distracted are encouraged to use the amino anxiety formula – tryptophan, histidine, glycine and taurine – to help them. Because of the calming effects of each member of the blend nutritionists and psychologists are using it increasingly simply to help people relax. Tryptophan, for example, can calm your mind approximately forty-five minutes after you take it. It is the precursor of vitamin B3 and serotonin, both important in maintaining the mental balance between activity and rest.

Histidine (as the precursor of histamine) will help to reduce the intensity of the excitory beta waves in the brain. The beta waves dominate when the body is under stress. On the other hand, the alpha waves, which histamine encourages, promote the relaxing body-at-rest functions of the parasympathetic nervous system.

Glycine and taurine in turn each help to calm the involuntary physical agitation of stress. For the full formula see page 66.

The mind-relaxing effects of meditation or biofeedback coupled with the remarkable synergistic powers of the amino formulas will help to heighten your resistance to infection. In turn, this reduces your chances of catching herpes. And if you have already been infected by the virus, controlling your stress in this way will help to inhibit the possibilities of further outbreaks. But raising your stress-threshold in this way is very much a long-term prevention programme. There is one herpes treatment, however, which is being used dramatically and effectively against the virus: the essential amino acid lysine.

Wonder-Working Lysine

The possibility of using lysine to combat herpes has been explored since the early fifties. One particularly important piece of research was conducted by an American, Dr R. Tankersley. Working with a herpes virus growing in a culture dish, he found that the addition of arginine – an essential amino for the production of growth hormone – stimulated the virus. However, when he added the structurally similar amino, lysine, the virus' growth was severely inhibited. Following this discovery, high doses of lysine were given to forty-five herpes victims. Of these, forty-three showed an astonishing improvement. The vesicles on their skin faded much more rapidly than normal and the pain was nowhere near as great. While they continued to take the lysine no new lesions and blisters appeared. Lysine's effectiveness in treating the symptoms of herpes is now widely acknowledged. In the UK, for example, it is recommended by the Herpes Organization.

Arginine, on the other hand, actively encourages the growth of the virus. Remember that structurally arginine and lysine are very similar. Scientists believe that lysine's effectiveness is due to the virus confusing it for arginine. This is one of the luckiest cases of mistaken identity in modern medicine.

In order to suppress the virus in your body the arginine/lysine ratio must be high in lysine's favour. During the active outbreaks of herpes lesions you might take up to 1000 mg of lysine three times a day. This will help ease the pain and speed up the disappearance of the sores. You must be careful, though, not to deplete the arginine levels. Arginine is one of the most important amino acids and, during the growth period (until you are about 30), it cannot be made by the body. Inducing arginine deficiency by taking too much of the competing lysine may actually harm your immune response and increase your chances of developing arterial sclerosis. Once the initial herpes outbreak diminishes try and reduce your lysine dosage. Take perhaps 500 to 1000 mg a day to keep the dormant virus in check instead of the original 3000 mg. Better still, lysine can be bought as a cream. Simple apply it straight on the affected areas.

As well as the free-form powder or the cream, try to eat foods with a high lysine to arginine ratio. These include fish, chicken, beef and lamb, milk, cheese sprouts, beans and most fruit and vegetables. At the same time do your best to avoid the high arginine foods: gelatin, chocolate, carob, coconut, oats, wholewheat and white flour, peanuts and wheatgerm.

The Metabolic Meridian

We scarcely give the metabolic cycle of our body a second thought. But in this too we have a powerful weapon in the fight against herpes. As we saw in Chapter 8, the body's metabolic cycle is composed of two opposing phases: anabolic and catabolic. Once we know how these processes affect us we can manipulate them into literally tearing the herpes infection down.

The anabolic and catabolic processes, you may remember, make up the continuous bodily cycle of life, death and rebirth. When we are in an anabolic state our bodies are growing and regenerating. Tissue repair, wound healing and muscle build-up all happen anabolically. But at the same time aspects of this part of the life cycle can also be harmful to the body. The growth of cancer tumours, the build-up of plaque in the blood and the formation of moles and warts are also anabolic in nature.

When your body attempts to tear down part of the body – getting rid of dead blood cells, for example – it enters the destructive, catabolic, stage. This is every bit as important as its anabolic counterpart. For example the formation of antibodies to destroy tumours and infections is a catabolic process. And, like the anabolic period, it also has its harmful aspects. Muscle-wasting diseases such as muscular dystrophy are catabolic.

All the body's metabolic activity falls into one of these two phases. The formation of a blood clot is a building activity, so it is anabolic. Then, during a catabolic cycle the body attacks the clot to break it down. However, if for some reason the body becomes stuck in its anabolic phase the clot won't be broken down. It might even grow until it seriously endangers the body, leading to a heart attack or haemorrhage.

A healthy body undergoes a balanced daily anabolic/catabolic cycle – anabolic from around 4 am to 10 am then catabolic at about 4 pm until 10 pm, with a transitional state in between. However, many people's metabolism is predominantly one or the other. This imbalance allows a variety of illnesses to attack and overcome the body. We've seen how an anabolic body lets the blood clot grow until it becomes dangerous. The same thing happens with herpes, because the attack that the herpes virus mounts on the body – both in the nerve cells and on the skin surface – is a building-up process. It is anabolic. Therefore, if we can find a way of tilting the biochemical balance of your body in favour of the catabolic phase we can actually counter the anabolic attack of the virus. But how? There's surely no such thing as 'free-form catabolic powders'. Well in a way, thanks to the research of Dr Emanuel Revici, there is.

Revici found that, depending on their electrical charge, some chemical elements behave anabolically and others catabolically. Experimenting with food molecules derived from these elements, he realized that they retained their anabolic or catabolic effect. When he gave these foods to patients whose metabolic balance was disrupted he was able to restore their normal anabolic/catabolic cycles.

All amino acids are either anabolic or catabolic. In fact, because they promote growth and regeneration most of them are anabolic. Some, however, do behave catabolically and we can use them to treat the herpes virus. They are methionine, cysteine, taurine, asparagine and glutamic acid. Taken in a blend they can actively inhibit the growth of the infection. Assisting the body's own catabolically based defences, they will help it to tear down the viral inflammation when it occurs. A catabolic formula might look like this:

Aminos
methionine
cysteine

taurine
aspartic acid
glutamic acid

Co-factors
A
B6
B12
folic acid
C as calcium ascorbate
magnesium aspartate
For maximum benefit try to take this formula in the early evening at
the start of your catabolic cycle.

We've listed several methods for controlling the effects of herpes.
But do they work? For the answer let's look at the case of Alastair, a
teacher who came to us not long ago in desperation. He had suffered
a rash of painful sores some years before which had been diagnosed
by his doctor as fungal growth. As the rash disappeared following a
short course of antibiotics he had no reason to question the doctor's
opinion. Recently he became engaged. Amid the chaos and stress of
moving to a larger house and making their marriage arrangements
the rash reappeared. His fiancée immediately contracted it,
suffering unbearable vaginal pain as a result. It was so debilitating,
in fact, that she was forced to take time off work. 'I realized straight
away it was herpes,' said Alastair, 'We both had it really badly. It
was as if our skin had been scraped raw and set on fire. Everyone I
spoke to said there was nothing we could do, that we just had to live
with it.' Determined not to accept this, he came for nutritional
counselling.

Urinary amino tests showed that they were both suffering from
dangerously low amino acid levels almost across the board. 'There
was so much to think about with the wedding and everything. We
were both eating out of tins and under a hell of a lot of stress.'
Accordingly, both he and his wife were put on the full stress control
programme and prescribed high doses of supplemental lysine.
While the agonizing lesions persisted they also took the catabolic
amino formula to help break the sores down.

The symptoms faded for both of them within forty-eight hours. 'I
can't begin to describe the immense relief we felt,' he said later. 'It
made life seem twice as great.' What it has also done is to show
Alastair and his wife how important a healthy, nutritionally
balanced lifestyle is, regardless of whether they are threatened by
illness or not. Because if you want to contain your herpes you need a

healthy body. Your digestion must be in good shape; you must be mentally stable and you must be able to withstand stress without your metabolic pathways becoming depleted of nutrients. Natural vitality is the best weapon you can possibly have in fighting the virus. Without doubt, the free metabolic energy of amino acids represents the best way of achieving that vitality.

General Wellbeing

Amino acids are the shock troops in the fight against herpes, but even they need logistical support. Make sure your gut has enough of the lactobaccilli, acidopholus and biffidus – the bacteria which are important for healthy digestion. They help break down the nutrients which the body needs for its stress response. They prevent allergic reactions from occuring in the gut, as well as fighting the bowel-related mood disorders. You can find these baccilli in foods like yoghurt and buttermilk or as tablet supplements. Zinc is also important for digestion. You need it for the formation of over eighty enzymes and many of these are in the stomach. It also helps your food to be fully absorbed.

Eat as much fresh food as you can, especially fruit and vegetables. Try to get most of your fibre from these sources rather than from bran which can easily irritate the gut. Cut out as much carbohydrate as you can, and don't eat any refined food.

Finally, make sure you get sufficient vitamin C. This has so many roles in the body, from helping to build collagen to the infection-fighting protein interferon. The body needs it everywhere and any small imbalance quickly creates stresses – particularly in your immune response.

Above all, don't be a helpless sufferer. The shock and stigma that people feel when they find they have herpes is enormous. It makes some withdraw from the human contact they need. Others try to boast about it as if they were wearing the latest Paris fashions. Neither of these attitudes is helpful. It's not a fashion or a cross to be borne but something you have to fight, actively and positively. If your life is stressful, if you eat poorly and rarely exercise you are much more likely to contract it – or endure greater suffering if you have it already. If, on the other hand, your lifestyle is healthy and balanced then you already possess the best defence against herpes that we know of, so go on, assert yourself.

Chapter 12

Allergy Answers

Most people are only dimly aware of how allergies affect them. Some know from experience to dread the start of summer and the inevitable attack of hayfever – with its blazing months of headaches, watery eyes and stuffy noses. Others are prevented from visiting a friend because of an allergy they may have to cat or dog fur. Beyond these common examples, though, the general knowledge and understanding of allergies is almost non-existent. Yet in reality there is an enormous variety of substances to which we are allergic. Tobacco smoke, for example, causes a reaction in almost everybody; many people can't drink milk or eat wheat without becoming ill and numerous pollutants and chemicals are continually affecting us – all without us realizing. How often do you have a 'low day', physically drained and mentally sluggish, unable to eat without feeling queasy, perhaps with a little trouble breathing? What about the sores and ulcers in your mouth? Or the rash of dry, flaky skin on the back of your arms? These are all symptoms of allergies. In fact, if you suffer from rheumatoid arthritis there is a good chance that this too is caused by an allergy.

An allergy is an abnormally heightened sensitivity to a substance (allergen) which is brought into contact with the body. The traditional view that this sensitivity can be traced back to a single cause and steps taken to either avoid it or 'densensitize' your body to it is obsolete. There is such an incredible number of allergens that in many people allergic reactions occur continually. A radical new approach is needed, that strengthens the body's entire metabolism and in doing so mitigates its allergy-causing hypersensitivity. Over the past few years amino acids have been used in this way with astonishing success. They attack the causes of allergies at their roots. By improving your digestion, removing the hazards of damage-causing agents such as free radicals and balancing the resources of your body's immune system they offer the best way forward for literally millions of allergy sufferers.

Peptide Problems

The first allergy we'll look at is caused by the body's basic sensitivity to undigested protein. We've seen how the protein we eat must be broken down in the gut before being absorbed. Occasionally, however, protein chains manage to seep through the gut wall intact. The allergic response this causes – the reddening, swelling and flushing in the skin, for instance – occurs after the protein comes into contact with highly sensitive tissue hormones called kinins. This happens because the kinins, activated by the protein, respond by tearing down the walls of neighbouring mast cells to release the substances contained inside – histamine, serotonin and heparin. Histamine, in particular, creates symptoms which range from mild fatigue, watery eyes or a blocked-up nose, to painful, suppurating rashes and aching muscles. It may lower your blood pressure, restrict the movement of blood and cause smoother, slower muscle contractions. Sore back muscles and the difficulty that asthmatics have in inhaling is often caused by this constrictive process.

Mast cells are confined mainly to the skin surface, but the kinins' response to protein can occur anywhere in the body. The inflammation they cause can be particularly harmful if it happens around the nerves. Kinin inflammation can even affect the brain, leading to headaches, migraine, nausea and lethargy. In extreme cases experts have found that it will even cause schizophrenia.

Remember, all these are all symptoms of the body's allergy to foreign proteins. But how are these foreign proteins able to enter the body in the first place? The answer lies in the simple inability of many people to digest their food. To function effectively our digestion must have sufficient stomach acid and a variety of amino-derived proteolytic enzymes, as well as controlled colonies of bacteria and yeast. If the digestive process falters in any way (perhaps as a result of inadequate stomach acid or simply from eating too much protein) fewer of the essential nutrients in your food will be released. This can lower the availability of the fresh amino acid sources which your pancreas needs for creating its enzymes. As a result, the levels of enzyme secretions drop, even less food is digested, and the domino-like destructive pattern is set in motion.

As we've just seen, allergies are one of the first results of this destructive process. Without the proteolytic enzymes needed to break the protein chains down into their constituent amino acids, the peptides either sit in the gut and putrefy or begin to seep through the intestine wall. Once this happens they are quickly absorbed into the blood. The blood's circulatory system distributes food so efficiently that the offending peptides which escape from the gut will soon come into contact with the kinins, reacting almost anywhere in the body. As well as the kinin and mast cell reactions, the gut wall itself often responds to contact with these renegade proteins by secreting an extra layer of mucus to protect itself. This causes a lubricating effect and often leads to diarrhoea.

Peptide Protection

When their sinuses start hurting, or when they suffer an asthma attack, few people imagine that the blame might lie with their digestion. Instead they try to relieve the symptoms by taking a man-made antidepressant or an anti-inflammatory synthetic hormone. Sometimes they might turn to plain and simple aspirin. Yet the side-effects of these substances are often worse than the disorder. Antidepressants, for example, artificially stimulate the body into producing noradrenalin, blocking the natural metabolic pathway from phenylalanine to adrenalin in the process. The stress which this puts on the pathway often leads to shortages of intermediate substances like the inhibitory L-dopa. This in turn frequently causes chronic illnesses, such as motor and mood disorders and clinical diabetes. Synthetic hormones, on the other hand, some-times undermine the activity of the endocrine system, waste the calcium in your bones and cause osteoporosis. Even aspirin may cause intestinal haemorrhaging – and, with digestion the cornerstone of your health, this is the very last thing you want.

Rather than suppressing these allergy symptoms, which is what conventional drug therapy is best at, amino acids work by attacking the causes of the allergies. Let's see what kind of formula you can use to prevent peptide seepage. First, if your stomach acid levels need raising you can include supplements of glutamic acid HCL and histidine in your diet. The ability of these aminos to stimulate stomach acid release and raise the levels of pepsin, the stomach enzyme, has been proved many times in the last decade. Glutamic acid also helps to ease the stresses on the pancreas – the gland which manufactures all the proteolytic enzymes. Two enzymes are especially important – chymotrypsin and carboxypeptase – as they work by reducing inflammation caused by the kinins. Every enzyme is vital for thorough digestion; to ensure that the pancreas has all the necessary raw materials for its job, you should also include in your formula a supplement of the complete amino acid blend. Finally, to raise you from the allergy-induced torpor take phenylalanine. As the precursor of adrenalin and noradrenalin it helps to stimulate you physically and mentally. So your peptide protection formula should look something like this:

Aminos
complete blend
glutamic acid HCL
histidine
phenylalanine   (not to be included if you also take MAO inhibitors, see p. 192)

Co-factors
B3
B6
C

Mechanics of Immunity

Of course, if undigested protein were the only cause of allergies life would be much easier than it is. In fact, the number of allergens with which we come into contact is almost unlimited. It includes drugs, pollen and moulds, animal fur, dandruff, bacteria, many different foods, smoke and pollution. Depending on how they contact the body – either by ingestion in the gut or the lungs, or absorbed through the skin – they may cause fever, rashes, diarrhoea, headaches and arthritis. The only characteristic that all allergies have in common is the abnormal, hypersensitive reaction they cause.

At the root of this response is the thymus gland, responsible for your immunity from invaders such as virus infections. We saw in chapter 8 how it guards against attacks from foreign substances by secreting a hormone called thymosin. This hormone orders the spleen and the lymph nodes to produce defences against the substance – T-cells and B-cells. Let's look at them a little more closely.

B-cells, also known as antibodies, are amino acid structures which unite with the invading allergen to render it harmless. If the allergen is a toxin the antibody neutralizes it. If it is bacteria the antibody coats it like a second skin, insulating it from the threatened tissue. If the allergen happens to be a virus the antibody blocks the attachment points between it and the cell it is trying to infect. Collectively, antibodies are called the immunoglobins (Ig) and this grouping is split into five smaller groups – A,D,E,G and M.

Each group performs a different role in the immune system. All the IgM antibodies, for example, are responsible for neutralizing toxins. Because of the way their connecting sites – the area on the surface of the antibody which makes contact with the invader – are structured antibodies are very selective, but not quite exclusive, about what they attack.

Now let's look at the other branch of the immune system, the T-cells. These are divided into several groups – lymphocyte, lymphokine and macrophage, as well as helper and suppressor cells. Lymphokines, the body's natural drugs, are responsible for the rashes which result from contact with allergens such as poison ivy. As well as working on their own T-cells, they also cooperate with B-cell antibodies. When T-cells meet an invader the number of helper cells compared to suppressor cells increases. This in turn raises the number of antibodies present to fight the allergen. Conversely, suppressor cells literally 'suppress' the rate of antibody production. So when we examine the number of circulating T-cells the overall total isn't the only important figure. The balance between helpers and suppressors matters as well. Because if the number of helpers constantly outweighs the suppressors your immune system will become oversensitive and allergic reactions will start to occur.

Auto-immune Excesses

Most allergies can be traced back to two related sources. The first is that the immune systems of as many as one person in ten produce more T-cell helpers than suppressors. These helper cells lead to the formation of increased numbers of antibodies – even though there may be no dangerous invading substances in the body. If these antibodies reacted exclusively to the substances which they were designed to fight this overproduction would be harmless. But, because invading substances change – viruses, for example, are constantly altering their structures – the defending antibodies must also be able to adapt in order to be effective. For this to happen the structures of their connecting sites allow for a certain latitude in what they latch on to. So when their numbers are abnormally increased by T-cell helpers, and in the absence of any harmful substances for them to attack, the antibodies might turn on almost anything as an invader. The result will be the symptoms of an immune response – headache, inflammation, fever – as the antibodies start reacting to the most innocuous, everyday substances: dust, pollen, foods and even the body's own tissue.

The second related cause of this allergy response is the IgE group of antibodies. As its main purpose is to fight parasitic diseases, IgE has become almost redundant in developed countries. During an abnormal increase in T-cell helpers, IgE fixes itself to the histamine-containing mast cells. When it encounters an allergen (as distinct from a substance which might actually be dangerous to the body) it breaks open the cell wall, spilling the contents. This leads to the familiar symptoms of sneezing, runny nose and inflammation – called 'atopy' – that we've already looked at. So how can we use amino acids to treat these antibody responses?

One of the most effective forms of allergy relief is supplemental histidine. As well as the invaluable help which this amino gives victims by stimulating stomach acid secretion, histidine also works in another way. In the case of atopy it has the ability to regulate the ratio of helper cell to suppressor. This is a little surprising as its amine form, histamine, is a central component of the allergy response – the flushing and inflammation. Histidine's suppressor/ helper balancing action actively prevents an allergic response from occurring. Histidine supplementation can unblock nasal passages and resolve redness and swelling. Furthermore, the irritability, depression or anxiety which often accompany an allergy response are also relieved.

When Steven, a bookseller, first came for nutritional counselling he was suffering from hayfever, although he looked more like the losing contender of a boxing match. His eyes were as swollen as lemons, his nose was a livid mauve, streaming constantly, and he spoke with a slurred, asthmatic wheeze. Rather than carrying out the usual tests, he was advised to take 500 mg of supplemental histidine three times a day for an initial two weeks, before deciding on a fuller course of treatment. He telephoned less than a week later to say that he wouldn't be visiting again as his symptoms had completely disappeared. Listening to him speak, in a voice that gave no hint of asthma or inflammation, it was hard to believe he was the same person.

When it comes to mitigating allergic responses histidine is one of the best aminos you can take. But what is it that initially causes the body to create more helper cells than suppressors and how can we remedy it? For the answer let's pay a visit to the free radicals.

Radical Policies

Free radicals are one of the most dangerous threats to your body's health. Very simply, free radicals are unstable molecules which carry an unpaired electron. Excessive levels of heavy metals in the air or your food leads to the creation of free radicals. Radiation and ultra-violet light create free radicals, as does any sort of illness or injury to tissue. A free radical's only goal in life is to find another electron to balance its atomic charge. It will stop at nothing to get it. Plundering the protein structures of your body in its search, it oxidizes cells, causing inflammation, injury and destruction. As we'll see in chapter 15, free radical damage is one of the main causes of ageing – it forms cross-links of damaged tissue in the structure of collagen so that your skin loses its resiliency, becoming wrinkled and leathery. And it raises the toxicity levels in your body so that the immune system comes under greater stress.

Free radical activity in fats creates dangerous peroxides. You can tell this yourself by smelling butter which has been left for too long and has become rancid. Free-radical-generated rancidity also occurs in the essential unsaturated fatty acids of your body and is one of the major causes of increased helper cell activity. Let's see why.

Basically, the peroxides which result from free radical activity work as blocking agents. They prevent a substance in the fatty acids from metabolizing to a short-lived regulating molecule called prostoglandin E1 (PGE1). It is PGE1 which stimulates the function of the T-cell suppressors. Without it the T-cell ratio is disrupted and, as we've seen, the body becomes hypersensitive to a variety of harmless substances.

PGE1 is converted in four stages from a component in the essential fatty acids called linoleic acid. The first stage of the transformation pathway converts linoleic acid to gamma-linoleic acid, and it is this conversion which the free radicals prevent. This can lead not only to common food allergies and a sensitivity to fur and pollen, but also to the auto-immune diseases such as rheumatoid arthritis. How can we protect ourselves from free radical damage? One answer is with glutathione.

Glutathione is a tripeptide. This means that it's made from three other amino acids – cysteine, glutamic acid and glycine. In the body glutathione combines with the mineral selenium to produce an enzyme called glutathione synthase. Tests have shown that using glutathione to increase the levels of this enzyme in the body prove remarkably successful in helping to relieve allergic responses. Acting as a 'free radical scavenger', glutathione synthase helps prevent the formation of fatty acid peroxides. This, in turn, allows the metabolism of PGE1 to occur normally.

As it works on all auto-immune illnesses, glutathione can help to reduce the inflammation, tissue degeneration and pain of rheumatoid arthritis. It is also an excellent chelator, removing from the body dangerous accumulations of heavy metals such as cadmium and lead – themselves free radical sources. It is even being used experimentally to clear up various airborne pollutants such as factory smoke, chemicals and bacteria from lung tissue. All these substances are major causes of allergies. Before long we might be using glutathione to treat allergies caused by anything from car fumes to pollen, milk and even the gluten in wheat.

As glutathione is a tripeptide, taking it as a complete supplement means that much of it might be broken down by the proteolytic enzymes in the gut. Glutathione is also a very expensive supplement. Instead of taking it in a complete dose, many people prefer to take a blend of its three constituent aminos, together with selenium. These aminos act as a base from which your body can manufacture glutathione. A good anti-allergy blend would look something like this:

Aminos
glycine
cysteine
glutamic acid
You can also add histidine.

Co-factors
selenium
B6
C

Allergies are one of today's major health problems. Some experts in the field even insist that every single illness, from arthritis to cancer, is allergy-related. Whether this is true or not, much of the conventional allergy therapy has tended to treat the obvious symptoms rather than attempt to come to grips with the deeper causes. Even some of the most respected forms of therapy currently available deal with individual allergies instead of questioning why a patient should be allergic to particular substances in the first place. Now, thanks to amino-based nutritional therapy, we can truly start to combat the fundamental causes of allergy.

Chapter 13

The Amino Slimming Revolution

Carefully selected blends of amino acid supplements make probably the most effective and versatile aids to weight reduction you'll ever find. Most diet programmes, while stressing how they will reshape your figure, completely ignore the damage they can cause to the body's hair-trigger-sensitive metabolism. As Richard Passwater says in his book, *Supernutrition for a Healthy Diet*, 'Most people diet not because they are overnourished, but because they are overfed.' Making sure that the body is adequately nourished while dieting is a concern that rarely enters the slimming equation. The slimming programmes offered by amino acids are quite different.

Although every cell in your body needs a stable and complete supply of nutrients this fact is actively ignored by many magazines columns on diet, and faddish health manuals. Passed on to the would-be dieter, the ignorance can lead to fatigue, a suppressed immune system, malnutrition, a variety of emotional disorders and sometimes anorexia. Often, ironically, it causes a metabolic backlash which might actually make you gain weight. By criticizing those diets we're not saying that if you are overweight you should stay that way. You only have to look at people a mere ten pounds over their ideal weight to realize how unhealthy it is: dandruff and dental decay is much more common, the risk of developing varicose veins is higher and stress is much more prevalent. If you are overweight the need to diet isn't in question. What matters is that, as you slim, you live at the peak of health and mental awareness – not in some physical twilight world of fatigue and irritation.

Used to form part of a healthy, reducing diet, naturally acting amino acids are perhaps the best slimming supplements you can choose. By making your body work more efficiently – metabolizing fat and improving muscle tone – their ability to help you lose weight is phenomenal. As the body's essential building blocks, they guard against malnutrition and energy loss. Rather than having to endure the typical slimming grind – the self-denial sustained only by guilt – the increased energy and vigour they release will make dieting an actual pleasure. Aminos can be used in a variety of ways to help you slim. Let's go through them one by one.

Stuffing the Habit

One of the most frequent excuses for being overweight is the habit of eating to help you relax or pass the time. At work, for example, you might have a small snack during your tea break. The physical ritual of unwrapping a bar of chocolate, putting it to your mouth and chewing it, is a convenient way of shifting your mental focus away from work. Many people smoke for the same reason; which is often why, if they give up, they substitute food for cigarettes and immediately gain weight.

We also use food as a psychological crutch to cope with anxiety. In our day-to-day lives we experience anxiety frequently – from the demands of a high-pressure job, or in anticipation of a driving test, even from fretting over the fate of a soap opera character. Anxiety is a sign of our bodies reacting to a situation by firing the sympathetic nervous system. Eating a snack in these situations is an unconscious attempt to engage the parasympathetic nervous system and restore the autonomic balance. As you chew, and as food passes down into the stomach, digestive enzymes are secreted, blood is pumped away from the heavy muscles, and brainwave activity slows. This helps to relieve the physical sensations of anxiety. For proof, look at cinema statistics. They show that audiences of horror films invariably eat the most popcorn and confectionary.

The compulsion to eat when you don't really want to – out of habit or in response to anxiety – is the first problem to tackle when you slim. So to help you start your diet try using the amino anxiety formula. Taken mid-morning and mid-after-noon (about two hours after breakfast and lunch respectively) the formula helps relieve the anxiety and tension which force you to eat. Many slimmers also find that it improves their overall performance at work, enhancing their concentration and improving their physical coordination.

Say No More

Many nutritionists and dieters agree that phenylalanine is the most effective slimming amino of all. This is because it is the parent molecule of three different metabolic pathways, all of which affect your weight. The benefits to your body of stimulating each of these pathways tend to overlap and strengthen the others. In two cases phenylalanine works by helping to curb your appetite. In the third it ensures that the food you do eat is used constructively by the body for cell growth and energy rather than accumulating as fat. This one amino is practically a weight reduction programme on its own.

Let's first look at how it curbs your appetite. Experts have recently found that phenylalanine triggers the release in your stomach of a substance called cholycystokinin (CCK). As far as appetite is concerned, CCK is a hormonal dipstick. When your stomach is empty CCK levels tend to be very low. This relays a message to the brain, telling you that the body needs food, which you experience as familiar hunger pangs.

Within half an hour of consuming a large meal, the levels of CCK in your stomach have risen by around 50 per cent. The new, higher level tells the brain that your body has eaten enough and, as a result, makes you feel physically sated. When you reluctantly refuse that third helping of chocolate mousse at a dinner party your CCK levels are at their highest. Using phenylalanine supplements to induce CCK release is the perfect way of cutting down the amount of food you eat. Taken last thing at night many people find that it helps them to avoid those nutritionally worthless, but fattening, mid-morning and mid-afternoon snacks, as well as choosing smaller helpings at mealtimes. Unlike the anxiety blend, which strengthens your mental resolve not to eat, phenylalanine is effective because it makes you feel physically full.

The second appetite-curbing pathway involves phenylalanine's conversion to noradrenalin. This excitory neurotransmitter – which is used widely to treat depression – elevates your mood, and quite simply, reduces your desire to eat. The active chemicals in prescribed appetite suppressant drugs, amphetamines, also work by releasing noradrenalin. But amphetamines prevent its reabsorption after use which can seriously deplete this important neurotransmitter. Some people on these drugs have actually become anorexic as a result of noradrenalin deficiency. Phenylalanine works differently. It allows for the natural reabsorption of noradrenalin into the nerve cells. It curbs appetite, and leaves you feeling energetic and positive with none of the dangerous side-effects. Try 250 mg of phenylalanine three times a day (mid-morning, mid-afternoon and just before bed), together with the vitamin co-factors of B6 (50 mg) and C (750 mg). There is just one warning: you should avoid using phenylalanine if you are already taking MAO inhibitors (see p. 192).

The amino Alamo

The third benefit of phenylalanine to your weight reduction programme comes from its role as the precursor of the amino acid tyrosine. Tyrosine helps your body to stay at its desired weight once you reach it. This is a godsend for the thousands of dieters who find that staying slim is even harder than losing weight in the first place. Exactly why is it so difficult, and how can tyrosine help? Well, let's imagine that by reducing your calorie intake you've lost every ounce you set out to lose. You naturally feel delighted. Within weeks, though, the jubilation vanishes as your body inexorably starts to regain the weight it shed.

The responsibility for this disheartening, and very common, reversal lies with the thyroid gland – one of the endocrine organs that controls the body's metabolism rate. By secreting the hormone thyroxin it dictates the extent of generation and growth of every cell in the body, as well as the amount of food which is burnt as energy. To the thyroid gland your sudden calorie reduction is the equivalent of an army raising a siege. In a siege, the attacking army attempts to starve the defending inhabitants into submission. And in resisting, the inhabitants must conserve as much of their food as they can. Your body is exactly the same. To prolong the existing supplies of food the thyroid gland secretes less thyroxin and this reduces the energy-burning metabolism rate. The fact that energy is conserved instead of burnt is one reason why you get so tired when you diet.

Several weeks pass. Standing on your bathroom scales you find you've reached your target. Not wanting to shed any more weight, you relax your eating habits a little. To the embattled thyroid gland the additional food is welcome, but it has no way of knowing whether this food signals an end of the siege or merely a lull between assaults. So rather than secreting more thyroxin to raise the metabolism rate – which will burn the food as energy and increase cell regeneration – the thyroid cunningly maintains the low rate, making the body hoard the food as insurance against further siege. Stored in the body and doing nothing, the food quickly turns to fat, resulting in your dismaying weight increase.

The key to all this is the mischief caused by the low thyroxin levels. Taking it one step further, if you were to raise the amount of thyroxin circulating in the body – so increasing the metabolism rate – the food you ate would be used to release energy and generate cell repair, rather than accumulating as unwanted fat. This is where tyrosine comes in. For it is this molecule which, combining with iodine in the thyroid gland, produces thyroxin. Supplementing the

117

amount of tyrosine in your body together with iodine, vitamin B6 and vitamin C will provide the materials to raise the natural thyroxin levels. Taken three times a day – mid-morning, mid-afternoon and before going to bed – they give your body the support it needs to metabolize your food instead of letting it sit as unwanted ballast.

Feeding the Furnaces

Carnitine is another amino acid attracting attention for the way it prevents fat from building up. Research into the way our bodies use carnitine shows that it metabolizes fat deposits in the blood vessels and muscles. Having broken down these formations of fat into fatty acids carnitine carries them into the cells and across the membranes of the mitochondria – minute cell engines which enable the body to utilize its food properly – where they are burnt as fuel. Urinary amino tests show that the carnitine levels of overweight patients are very low. As a result they suffer from high blood cholesterol levels and often from high blood pressure. When the same patients are given a course of supplemental carnitine their cholesterol levels show a dramatic drop, frequently blood pressure is eased and weight loss becomes much easier to achieve.

The energy which is released when the fatty acids are burnt also has other benefits. It can lead to increased alertness, greater stamina and heightened sexual interest. Considering the periods of fatigue that dieters are usually forced to endure, the free energy provided by carnitine is further proof of the advantages of using amino acids.

Carnitine also protects dieters from ketosis. This is the damage caused by an accumulation of ketone bodies – the toxic waste products of fat. Ketones are left behind like sediment in a wine bottle when fat is mobilized. They raise the level of acidity in your blood and make the body dump vital minerals such as potassium, calcium and magnesium. This can lead to kidney damage and may even be life-threatening if it continues uncontrolled; 250–500 mg daily of carnitine on an empty stomach will help to prevent it.

Battle of the Binge

A very popular method of weight reduction among slimmers today is a diet that consists almost exclusively of protein – with as little carbohydrate as possible. There is, however, a serious and largely unrecognized drawback to this, one that consistently drives would-be slimmers to binge foods with a high carbohydrate content such as biscuits and cakes. The cause of the problem lies in a link that connects the levels of tryptophan with the amount of carbohydrate we normally eat.

A tryptophan molecule is larger than any other amino acid. Yet most aminos are distributed throughout the body by the same pathways. This means that the large, cumbersome tryptophan must compete with smaller, nimbler aminos such as isoleucine and methionine for absorption – through the gut wall, across the blood brain barrier and wherever else it is needed. Its sheer size prevents it from being absorbed as thoroughly as the others. One of the immediate effects of your high protein meal, in which large numbers of amino acids 'jostle' for space, is that less tryptophan is able to reach your brain.

Unlike protein, carbohydrate will raise tryptophan levels in relation to the other aminos. This is because eating food with a high carbohydrate content increases the amount of sugar in your blood. The sugar in turn triggers an insulin release and this has the effect of diverting the circulating amino acids away from the brain – all, that is, except tryptophan. The tryptophan, unaffected by insulin, finds its path into the brain suddenly unblocked and enters with ease.

Keep this in mind if you decide to slim using a high protein, low carbohydrate diet. This diet will almost certainly work to depress your brain tryptophan levels – something which you should always try to avoid. Why is tryptophan so important? Primarily because it is the precursor of serotonin and when a high protein diet depletes tryptophan the level of this brain chemical drops too. In previous chapters we've seen that serotonin is a crucially important neurotransmitter. From the brain, its calming, inhibitory action spreads throughout the body, mitigating our response to stress, relieving depression and anxiety and improving digestion. Most important of all, we need serotonin to be able to sleep and for the way it promotes natural, rhythmic sleeping patterns. By reducing the available serotonin, a high protein diet works against this. Carbohydrate, on the other hand, simply by encouraging tryptophan pickup, helps to improve these functions.

Not surprisingly then, slimmers on a high protein diet, and low in brain tryptophan, become fixated by a craving for carbohydrate. This is a sign of the body attempting to increase its tryptophan levels. The physical and mental sensations it causes (aggravated by the lack of calming serotonin) can be as tantalizing, and agonizing, as withdrawal symptoms. For many people the impulse to binge becomes overwhelming. The guilt and self-recrimination that follow are meaningless in that first, resigned instant of cloying satisfaction when they bite into their doughnut or Danish pastry. Any resolve simply flies out of the window, together with their diet.

The simple and effective solution to this is to take supplemental tryptophan. If you are already taking the complete anxiety formula (see p. 66) add an extra 100 mg a day of tryptophan approximately forty-five minutes before your meals. If you're not taking the anxiety formula try 500 mg a day. Many dieters find that this is all they need to dispel the anxiety and acuteness of their cravings. The dosage is even more effective if you eat a slice of wholemeal bread with it to aid brain pick-up. Admittedly, bread is a major source of carbohydrate. However, if you compare it to the packet of chocolate digestive biscuits that one patient confessed to eating in half an hour a single slice won't seem such a difficult concession to make.

Another amino which slimmers are finding helpful is glycine. Glycine is the most commonly occurring amino acid in the body. Because of its relatively small structure it is used as a sort of cement filling in the spiral structure of collagen, giving this protein structure its resiliency. Urinary amino tests show that glycine levels in victims of obesity are consistently much lower than average. Significantly, glycine has a pleasant, sweet taste and some nutritionists think that a link exists between the 'sweet tooth' of overweight people and a glycine deficiency. Their craving for sweet things is very probably caused by the body's efforts to replace the missing glycine.

The help that glycine and tryptophan gave to Don shows how effective they could be in your diet. A divorcee, Don's eating habits were basically very good – lots of fresh salads, fish, eggs and some lean meat, together with plenty of exercise. His problem was that almost every night he would follow his nutritious main course with a huge bowl of freshly baked rice pudding. 'It had almost as much sugar in it as rice,' he said, 'and there was a hell of a lot of rice. It was funny, the more often I cooked it, the more I enjoyed it, savoured it. Cooking and eating it was a sort of ritual. If I went out or couldn't be bothered to cook it I might actually start fretting and fantasizing about it.' As he was entering middle age, the excess carbohydrate and cholesterol were making him put on weight dramatically.

When he came for nutritional counselling it was to find help for his weight which he felt was starting to interfere with his social life. He was also suffering from insomnia – a sign of how low his tryptophan/serotonin levels were. It wasn't until tests showed depleted levels of glycine as well as the expected tryptophan that his rice craving came to light. A blend of these two aminos was recommended together with vitamins B3, B6 and C. As he reported later: 'I went completely off the thought of those rice and sugar binges. It amazes me now looking at the size of the bowl that I could eat so much of what was obviously doing me so much harm. Hell, it's almost big enough to do the washing up in.' His weight dropped considerably and he's been fine since.

Muscle-Bound Aminos

Another method of weight reduction centres on the use of amino acids to produce human growth hormones. The terrific advantage of growth hormone release (GHR) is that, in addition to burning off your fat deposits, the hormone actually helps strengthen and tone your muscles. Several aminos are responsible for GHR. The most important are arginine and lysine.

Growth hormone – also called somatrophic hormone – is secreted by the pituitary gland. It controls the manufacture of protein, determining where and how amino acids will be used in your body. It is responsible for the growth of long bones, skin and organs, and helps to stimulate the immune system. Like carnitine, it inhibits the formation of fat, mobilizing existing fat stores as fatty acids and burning them for energy. Strenuous physical exercise which saturates the body with oxygen is one of the natural triggers of GHR, accounting for the superb muscle tone of many athletes. The levels of this hormone are highest in children which explains why they can eat so voraciously without getting fat.

Growth hormone secretion declines sharply when we are about thirty. This is one of the causes of muscle wasting and bone thinning that occurs as we age. In the bodies of people beyond their mid-thirties, most of the available growth hormone is used to aid wound-healing and sustain the effectiveness of the immune system. For most of us there is just not enough remaining to metabolize our fat deposits. This is why amino acid supplements are so important. Arginine and lysine actually increase the levels of growth hormone released from the pituitary. New muscle protein is created at the expense of fat, which is burnt as energy. Tensile strength of the structural protein collagen is also increased. This is particularly important to slimmers. Instead of your skin sagging as you lose weight, healthy collagen will help it to contract to your new shape, retaining its firmness and pliability.

Experts recommend a maximum dosage of 6000 mg each of arginine and lysine, together with 200 mg of vitamin B6 and 500 mg of vitamin B3. If you suffer from a viral infection like herpes the arginine may aggravate it. In this case try ornithine in its place.

Although this molecule is produced from arginine, clinical experiments indicate that it has no effect on viruses, yet works effectively in triggering GHR. The best time to take this formulation is just before going to bed. This is because natural growth hormone secretion usually occurs some ninety minutes after we fall asleep. As a good night's sleep is vital, you might also consider supplementing the blend with extra tryptophan to stimulate the sleep-inducing serotonin. Another important precaution to remember is that you should also take these aminos on an empty stomach. This is because GHR also triggers the release of insulin – a metabolic jackdaw, searching for, and storing, any amino acids, fats or blood sugar that it can find. If you eat immediately before taking the growth hormone aminos the insulin will store the food and, instead of losing weight, you might start to put it on.

Wielding the Metabolic Axe

Like insulin, the aminos which the body uses to manufacture growth hormone effect your body anabolically. This is to say the functions they perform are essentially related to growth, to building up and regenerating cell structure. As we've seen with herpes, where the growth of the virus is an anabolic process, the anabolic phase can be harmful as well as helpful. For example, as far as dieting is concerned, the anabolic process caused by insulin is harmful because it leads to the growth of fat deposits. On the other hand, in harnessing the potential of growth hormone – that is, by taking the aminos on an empty stomach, we can use the anabolic process, which improves the body's muscle tone and collagen, to tear down the fat deposits.

You can see the ambiguous nature of the anabolic/catabolic cycle clearly by looking at the ways it affects anorexics and victims of obesity. You would think, naturally enough, that the physical results of an anorexic's obsessive concern with weight reduction – virtually trying to 'tear down' her whole body – would be well and truly catabolic. Surprisingly it isn't. In a near total state of depletion an anorexic body wedges itself obstinately into a permanent anabolic state, simply as a method of self-preservation. Continuously building itself up with the few resources it has is the only way it can survive. It's rather like trying to stop an incoming tide by using a toy spade to build a sand wall – the only chance you have of preventing the water from sweeping the wall away is frantically to pile more and more sand on top.

While the physical emaciation of anorexia is characterized by an anabolic response, obesity – is brought about by the efforts of a fat body to stave off further weight gain, like a dam opening its sluice gate to prevent the water in its reservoir from overflowing. Most of the amino therapies we've looked into so far are anabolic (phenylalanine, tyrosine, tryptophan and the growth hormone aminos). To ensure that the body's own catabolic defences against weight gain are not disrupted there are specific aminos you can take to strengthen your catabolic response. These catabolically based aminos are methionine, taurine, cysteine, asparagine and glutamic acid (see pp. 103–4 for details). Using them to supplement your body at the start of its catabolic cycle – between 4 and 10 pm – they will help to tear down the fat you can't see in your blood vessels, muscles and organs, as well as the fat you can see, bulging over the elastic of your underwear.

By timing these metabolic phases properly you are practically introducing a shift system, or relay, of weight-reducing measures into your body. Once the catabolic demolition finishes the anabolic one will begin, spearheaded by the bedtime supplements of the growth hormone aminos.

The story of one young woman, Marian, who came to us at her wit's end illustrates the importance of a balanced anabolic/catabolic cycle. She explained that during a year of severe emotional strain – her father's death coinciding with the break-up of her marriage – she had turned to food for support. Very quickly she gained an alarming fifty pounds. Finally realizing the danger, she switched to a diet consisting almost exclusively of fresh fruit. Her body rapidly shed twenty pounds; then it stopped. 'It just wouldn't lose another ounce,' she said 'It's as if it was stuck.' What had actually happened was that her metabolic balance, knocked around like a pinball first one way by the weight gain then the other by the diet, had finally reacted. In an effort to stabilize the fluctuations of weight it had become permanently anabolic, arresting any further weight loss by continuously building up tissue to compensate. Marian was given a high dosage of the catabolic aminos to take at five o'clock every evening. During the day she took carnitine and before bed the growth hormone releasing aminos, arginine and lysine. Her weight began to drop again and within three months she was back to her original weight.

As Marian discovered, slimming is a battle of wits between you and your body. Even when you do start to lose weight there is always the danger of being outmanouvered by its hormonal responses. Despite your best efforts you might inexplicably start to regain the weight you lost or find yourself caught in an irresistible craving for some high calorie, high carbohydrate food. Instead of fighting a dreary war of attrition against these things accept them for what they are – signs that your choice of weight reduction is harming you – and take steps to put things right. This means first and foremost satisfying the nutritional demands of your body. Using amino acids and their co-factors helps you to avoid causing dangerous nutritional depletions when you diet. And by helping your body to work more efficiently – building new muscle, burning excess fat and helping to resist cravings – the assistance they give you might make you wonder how you ever got on without them.

Chapter 14

The Amino Answer to Heart Disease

A heart attack is a metabolic thunderbolt. Until the instant it strikes, its victim usually feels in excellent health. He might not drink, or even smoke. He might be as strong as a horse and exercise strenuously. Of course, he may admit that he occasionally gets very hot and unaccountably short of breath, but nothing really to worry about. Driving to work one morning he reaches for the gear stick to change down a gear. Suddenly his arm feels heavy as if the blood in it has turned to lead. He hardly has time to wonder what's wrong before a jolt of pain rattles it from shoulder to wrist and an incredible, relentless, vice-like grip crushes across his chest, stealing his breath. Out of the blue his heart has stopped beating. Even with today's medical expertise more than fifty per cent of deaths in Britain and America happen in this way.

The health and efficiency of your heart and circulatory system – more crucially than anything except your brain – depends on a balanced lifestyle. Unfortunately, because of the way we systematically abuse our bodies few of us enjoy this optimal lifestyle. Smoking and drinking of alcohol are obvious abuses. They rob the cells of oxygen and vitamins, raise the levels of toxicity in the body, damage our endocrine organs and lead to high blood pressure.

But your heart can be hurt just as seriously by other, far subtler, problems. Even if you don't smoke or drink, even though you exercise regularly and follow a low cholesterol diet you could still suffer a heart attack. A history of poor digestion or nutrition, emotional problems, stress, even inherited disabilities all make you vulnerable. If they lead to a deficiency in your body of only a small number of vital nutrients this might be all it takes. Over the years (and heart attacks don't usually occur until the victim is well into middle age) the effects of these deficiencies will grow like the falling pebble which eventually causes a landslide. If, for example, a molecule needed to create an enzyme is missing, the metabolic pathway that uses this enzyme will be converted much more slowly than it should be. This in turn will starve the body of other specific nutrients. In the end the deficiencies will become widespread and highly damaging – nowhere more so than your heart.

Heart attacks are usually attributed directly to cholesterol build-up. Even when this is the obvious cause, the fact that the victim's body is unable to break the cholesterol down efficiently points to widespread enzyme, vitamin and mineral deficiencies and not just to a fatty diet.

So treating heart problems isn't only a question of cutting out certain foods. You must actually increase your intake of the nutrients which supply your body's relevant metabolic pathways. We've seen how these miraculous processes take raw materials from your diet and create the chemicals which meet the body's precise metabolic needs. They also break down fat and ensure that your cells have enough oxygen. When doctors search for the cause of heart problems, though, these unique biochemical processes are ignored. Instead, they look to high technology to enforce a 'cure': sophisticated by-pass surgery costing tens of thousands of pounds; 'piggy-back' heart operations and pacemakers; lasers to burn out the debris from blocked arteries; and, most incredible of all, the mechanical replacement hearts connected from the chest by wires to an outside power source. Then, to make the body accept these things the patient is given high doses of toxic drugs to suppress the immune system, in turn making him more vulnerable to infection and disease. Isolating any illness from its relationship to the rest of the body like this runs completely against the orthomolecular approach to health. The emphasis seems to be on relieving the obvious symptoms of the disorder rather than on attempting to trace the wider imbalances which cause the problem.

Furthermore, general advice about the danger of a high cholesterol intake is given with little or no awareness of the way that fats really affect us. For example, we are often told to reduce the number of eggs we eat. Yet eggs are an invaluable source of many nutrients, including lecithin – which actually helps to regulate how our bodies use fat – and sulphur. The fear that eggs cause a large build-up of blood cholesterol now appears to be largely unfounded. Besides, the fat in our diets accounts for only 20 per cent of the total cholesterol amount in the body. The rest is manufactured in the liver from carbohydrate. Nutritionists such as Dr Carl Pfeiffer believe that reducing the cholesterol we eat only increases its production by the liver. This in turn may lead to even higher fat levels than normal.

We believe that focusing exclusively on fat as the cause of heart disease is wrong. Instead we should look at the whole body and the metabolic pathways which affect fat and protein metabolism.

When the body allows fat to accumulate – when the arteries harden and your blood pressure rises – it is a sign that for some reason these pathways are not working as they should. Amino acids and their co-factors are being used with increasing success to treat these heart problems. As the essential raw materials of your metabolic pathways, they work by repairing, and rebalancing, those damaged pathways which cause heart disease.

Moving Methionine

The first pathway we'll look at involves using the amino acid methionine to relieve ateriosclerosis. Put simply, a victim of ateriosclerosis suffers from a hardening of his arteries. The subsequent rise in blood pressure is caused as his heart, in meeting the demanding oxygen requirements of his body, has to work harder to force blood through rigid, constricted vessels. The intense stress this puts on his heart is one of the most common causes of eventual heart failure.

As the build-up of cholesterol, and other fat products, is one of the immediate causes of this hardening process most doctors attribute ateriosclerosis to the abundance of fatty foods in our diets. In fact, research conducted as long ago as 1906 identifies poor protein metabolism, rather than fat build-up, as the major cause, and in particular the blockage of a metabolic pathway involving methionine. Let's see what happens. In this pathway methionine is converted to the amino acid cystathione. As we've seen before, most metabolic pathways consist of a series of step-by-step changes which transform the parent molecule to the exact substance your body requires. At an intermediate stage of this cystathione-creating pathway, methionine becomes the amino acid homocysteine. This chemical is one of the causes of arteriosclerosis.

In a normal, nutritionally balanced body the entire pathway takes a split second to complete. Methionine becomes homo-cysteine, which in turn is instantly converted to cystathione. To convert homocysteine to cystathione the body calls on an enzyme called cystathione synthase (itself manufactured from a metabolic pathway involving several vitamins and amino acids). The incredible complexity and precision of our bodies is shown by the fact that cystathione synthase is created solely to convert homocysteine to cystathione. However, if any of the nutrients needed to manufacture this enzyme are missing the conversion process is arrested, leaving homocysteine to circulate freely in the body.

But why is homocysteine so dangerous? Basically, because it's an abrasive. Passing through your bloodstream, it scratches and scrapes away at the delicate arterial walls like molecular sandpaper. As well as causing the arteries to harden, the roughened areas it leaves also make ideal anchoring points for fatty acid and calcium phospholipid deposits.

In time the arteries lose their pliability and clog up. The space available for the blood to flow shrinks. Simply to maintain the blood's normal circulating rate (as much as sixteen inches a second in major arteries) your blood pressure rises. Your heart, pumping harder and more frequently, is working under severe stress and its efficiency is reduced. Consequently, less oxygen reaches the cells. Frequent breathlessness, abnormal perspiration and high heartbeat and pulse rate are common symptoms of this illness. If they're not recognized in time the victim may suffer a heart attack or a stroke.

Fortunately, by supplementing your diet with the specific amino acids and co-factors which convert methionine, all this could be avoided. The nutrients needed for the enzyme which completes the pathway are vitamin B6 and the amino acid serine. B6 is easily destroyed by heat and its levels in food drop sharply if cooked. When just this one substance is missing or depleted, let alone any others, the body simply won't be able to metabolize homocysteine to cystathione. Adding supplements of vitamin B6 and serine to your diet, on the other hand, provides your body with the materials it needs to make the enzyme and helps to remove the harmful levels of homocysteine from the blood.

In a healthy body homocysteine will also convert back to the parent molecule methionine. The substances the body must have to be able to do this include adequate amounts of existing methione, several enzymes – all amino based – and vitamin B12. Like B6, B12 needs a special mention. It is a large molecule and its absorption can only take place in a special section at the lower end of the small intestine. If you suffer from digestive disorders, resulting perhaps in diarrhoea, much of the B12 will simply pass straight through the body. In order to get through the gut wall it also has to be coated with a mucinous protein called the 'intrinsic factor', which itself depends on the presence of a variety of component amino acids. So even if you decide to take supplements of B12 your digestion must be healthy, in order to absorb them. The best way to ensure this is with a supplement of the complete amino acid blend – on top of the individual supplements. Easily absorbed, they help the pancreas to manufacture all the necessary digestive enzymes.

One final word on the importance of methionine in preventing cholesterol build-up: it can also manufacture choline. This is a regulating molecule which maintains a favourable ratio between low density lipids – protective, unsaturated fats – and high density lipids – the dangerous, plaque-causing fats. Insufficient choline is another cause of arterioschlerosis.

You can see that deficiencies anywhere in the body cause problems far and wide. The complexity is amazing. Rather than thinking of arterioschlerosis simply as the result of eating too much cholesterol, we must look at it as a symptom of complicated biochemical imbalances. It is the shock-waves which these imbalances send through the entire body which cause the condition. The way that amino acids and their co-factors can be used to relieve it shows how important a body-wide awareness of nutrition can be.

'Heart Burn' Amino Style

L-carnitine is another amino acid well worth including in any heart relief formula. A deficiency of this amino allows fat to build up in the arteries, starves the cells of oxygen and can lead to angina. Carnitine is made in the liver from lysine and methionine, but taking it as a free-form supplement ensures that your body gets a full, balanced supply. Your body uses carnitine to transport fatty acids into and out of the cells across the cellular membranes. When your body is carnitine deficient fat deposits are allowed to gather in the blood vessels. As we've seen, this will eventually clog your arteries and lead to higher blood pressure.

Normally when carnitine is transporting fats efficiently across into the cells they are burnt as fuel by the energy-releasing mitochondria. We can see how important the fat-burning relationship between carnitine and the mitochondria is by looking at the bodies of physically active people such as swimmers and athletes. Their carnitine levels are generally very high and the fat in their blood is mobilized far more efficiently and thoroughly than normal. At the same time the mitochondria in their cells use the extra oxygen which is pumped into their bodies by intense physical activity to burn these extra fats and meet the greater demands for energy. This is why physically fit people are usually so lean and why the oxygen demands created by aerobic exercise is so beneficial.

Conversely the smaller energy and oxygen requirements of sedentary people cause the number of mitochondria in their bodies actually to shrink. As a result less of the fat from their diets is burnt. This is why people who rarely excercise tend to have slack, flabby bodies and high cholesterol levels. A similar problem affects those people who suffer from low carnitine levels. Without carnitine to break it down the fat begins to clog dangerously in the artery walls. At the same time, with less fat to burn, the number of cell mitochondria will drop. This causes in turn a decline in the tissue's oxygen requirements.

Looking specifically at the heart, this loss of oxygen has the effect of starving it of fuel and preventing it from performing to its full potential. Consequently, when an increased supply of blood is needed by the body – it could be from something as simple as running for a bus – the heart, in trying to cope without sufficient oxygen to fuel its response, will react with an agonizing, cramp-like pain. This is one of the symptoms of angina and acts as a warning of worse problems to come.

Free-form carnitine supplements have the effect of dredging the blood vessels of fat, which is then carried to the mitochondria to be burnt as bonus energy for your heart. With this rising level of fat metabolism, the distribution of mitochondria will increase. All this leaves the heart able to perform more efficiently without subjecting it to undue stress.

Amino Heart Flush

Another highly beneficial amino acid is tryptophan. Research by a number of independent medical teams shows that regular dietary supplementation of just this one amino could prevent a staggering 15 per cent of the deaths caused by heart attacks! Its effectiveness lies in the metabolic pathway which leads to the manufacture of serotonin. As well as helping us to sleep more soundly, the neuro-inhibitory effects of this chemical also promote smoother, more regular muscle contractions throughout the body. This is important in preventing the heart spasms and racing heartbeat that often occur before a heart attack. It also helps to avoid the damage to the blood vessels of fibrillation, which if left unchecked can lead to plaque build-up, hardening of the arteries and raised blood pressure.

Including tryptophan in a blend with the other aminos we've looked at in this chapter helps to enhance the individual benefits of each of these supplements. The tryptophan and carnitine, for example, relieve the physical stresses on your heart – one by relaxing the muscle contraction, the other by feeding it more oxygen and energy. At the same time methionine and serine, by getting rid of the abrasive homocysteine, make it easier for carnitine to flush the fat build-up from the artery walls.

One final amino that you might like to add to the blend is histidine. Histamine, its highly active amine form, is a calming neurotransmitter. It is also the most important substance released from the mast cells – the structures responsible for the reddening and flushing of the immune system. The response is helpful in dealing with heart problems – particularly if you supplement the histidine with the niacin or nicotinic acid forms of B3 forms of vitamin B3. This is because B3 helps the mast cells to burst, releasing histamine into the body. Mast cell discharge leads to watery eyes, a reddening of the skin and unpleasant sensations of itchiness and burning. These are symptoms of histamine's dilatory action on the skin capillaries. Even though they may be uncomfortable, the effect of forcing more blood to the surface of the skin is to lower your overall blood pressure and relieve the stresses on your heart. The niacin and nicotinic acid forms of B3 also help to lower fat levels in the blood.

Earlier we referred to the image of a single falling pebble causing a landslide to explain how nutritional deficiency can lead to heart disease. Now imagine watching a film of this scene being played backwards. Boulders seem to fly up the hill to relodge in their original places. The number of moving rocks gradually diminishes. Finally, we watch the pebble which started everything come to rest at the summit. Every stone is now back in its rightful place. This is the way that amino therapy works to relieve heart problems. Rather than conventional medicine, which would simply try to put the pebble back at the top without considering the destruction that has resulted, these amino supplements work by rectifying the entire landslide – which in terms of your body means making sure that all the affected metabolic pathways are balanced and in harmony. Let's look at a good heart-relief formula:

Aminos
methionine
serine
tryptophan
histidine
complete blend

Co-factors
B3 (niacin or nicotinic acid)
B6
B12
pantothenic acid
folic acid

C
E
magnesium
zinc

The formula also highlights the necessity of including vitamin and mineral co-factors. They are quite simply as important to the way your body uses amino acid supplements as cement is in keeping the bricks of your house in place. Let's see why.

Several notable researchers have demonstrated that vitamin C is a key nutritional supplement in metabolizing cholesterol. Sherry Lewin, for example, found that sodium ascorbate (the mineral form of vitamin C) combines with molecules of the insoluble substance, calcium phospholipid. This chemical is one of the fat by-products that carnitine and methionine help to dislodge from the artery wall. Because of its insolubility it often circulates in the blood until it finds another resting place. Then it starts to accumulate all over again. However, when it meets with sodium ascorbate a chemical reaction creates calcium ascorbate and sodium phospholipid, both of which are soluble. In this way the body can easily eliminate the dangerous calcium phospholipid.

Vitamin C's ability to cleanse blood vessels is verified by Emil Ginter. Experimenting with guinea pigs (one of those rare animals which, like human beings, are unable to produce vitamin C) he found that a shortage of vitamin C caused their veins and arteries to clog. When he administered high doses of vitamin C supplements the blockages gradually cleared. Together with zinc, vitamin C is also an important structural component of blood vessels, helping to maintain their ability to dilate.

Vitamin E, on the other hand, gives structural flexibility to red blood cells. This stops undue clotting which in turn can lead to plaque build-up and eventual haemorrhaging. Vitamin E also prolongs the life of red blood cells and increases their oxygen-carrying capacity – immensely important in helping to reduce high blood pressure.

The Escape Claws

Another way of using amino acid supplements to treat heart problems is now receiving a lot of attention. This method is called chelation therapy. Chelation means literally to form a claw. The process involves using special molecules to search the body like metabolic bloodhounds for dangerous and toxic minerals. When they find them, the searchers grasp them like claws and the body is then able to eliminate the combined substances in the urine.

Of course, there are only a limited number of substances with specific structures which will chelate. The most effective are a small group of aminos headed by the versatile methionine. In addition to protecting blood vessels from fat build-up, methionine also acts as a chelator guarding against calcium deposits. Excessive amounts of calcium in the wall of the veins and arteries contribute to the hardening and fibrillation of arterioschlerosis. Methionine supplements help to prevent this.

Chelators also work against free radical activity. Free radicals you may remember are the electronically unstable molecules which, in their search for stability, attract electrons from other substances destroying them in the process. Pollutants, such as the heavy metals cadmium, copper and mercury, are recognized as causes of hypertension and arterioschlerosis in blood vessels and organs. Much of the research into the effects of free radical activity shows that the destruction they cause – ripping down cell membranes, oxidizing vitamins and neutralizing vital enzymes – leads to the formation of atherones (fatty plaques). As these build up in the blood vessels your blood pressure rises and the heart and other organs are starved of oxygen. Doctors and nutritionists agree that heavy metals are major causes of heart disease and strokes, yet with the high levels of pollution in our cities they seem unavoidable. Fortunately by using amino acids to chelate these substances we can avoid them.

As well as methionine, the amino acid cysteine is an excellent chelator. Together with glycine and glutamic acid, cysteine is also part of glutathione. This tripeptide is being used to chelate free radicals in a variety of illnesses including allergies, rheumatism and smoking complaints.

Finally some experts are starting to use the amino acid ethylene diametetranetic acid (EDTA), which is one of the most powerful chelators known. The problem with EDTA, which is the same to a lesser extent with all chelators, is that it isn't selective about which minerals it claws on to. An example of this is the way that EDTA is used commercially in the food processing industry. Scalding vegetables such as broccoli, peas and spinach with EDTA removes all heavy metals from their surfaces so that they appear lustrously green rather than their natural, greyer appearance. But when these vegetables are analysed not only are the levels of metals like chromium lower but also nutritious substances like zinc and manganese are found to be depleted to about 20 per cent of their normal levels. The same thing may happen with chelation therapy in the body. It's important to seek advice from a qualified doctor or nutritionist before using EDTA. They will monitor the mineral levels in your body and recommend specific nutrients should their levels drop.

So how do the supplements mentioned in this chapter work in practice? Let's find out by looking at a case history. Rob is a warehouseman in his mid-forties. His physically demanding job involves shifting crates that weigh up to a hundred pounds. He has never smoked, hardly drinks and is active in his spare time as well as at work. One day, unloading a truck, he felt a sharp, stabbing pain in his chest and a dull sensation in his legs, almost as if they had gone to sleep. Hospital tests showed that his arteries were severely hardened and clogged. 'The doctor said it was only because I was so strong and active that I hadn't had a heart attack,' Rob said. Unfortunately there was nothing the doctor could do to reverse the clogging process. He put Rob on a course of drugs designed to keep the symptoms at bay and told him to reduce his exertion at work. He was to come back in six months for a check-up when they would decide whether a by-pass operation was needed.

During the following months Rob's wife Michelle read about the benefits of amino testing and therapy. Anxious to try anything that might help him she made an appointment for her husband to come for nutritional counselling. After the usual tests he was first recommended the complete amino blend to stimulate the enzyme systems throughout his body. In addition, he was told to take a blend of the three aminos that form the chelator glutathione (cysteine, glutamic acid and glycine), as well as carnitine and methionine. The co-factors included vitamin B6, vitamin B complex, magnesium, manganese, zinc and sodium ascorbate (the mineral vitamin C). A few weeks later Michelle telephoned. 'Rob suddenly has so much energy,' she said, 'Is it alright if I take the formulation too? I won't be able to keep up with him otherwise.'

At the end of the six months Rob returned to his doctor for the check-up. 'He was so surprised,' Rob recalled, 'For a moment he thought he'd mixed up his case notes because my arteries were in such great shape. He said: "I don't know what you've been doing but keep it up."'

Chapter 15

Stay Young With the Free Aminos

Hidden in the shadows of a dank, unlit attic sits a portrait in oils. Moving downstairs we spy the subject of this painting, a young, handsome man perhaps in his late twenties. Engrossed in conversation with a friend, he speaks with the passion and vigour of his years. Yet although the face of the young man and the face in the portrait belong to one and the same person, the figure in the portrait is old. Its cheeks are haggard and pale and creased; thin wisps of hair sit limply on the forehead and folds of sallow skin sag from the throat. As with each passing year this face grows a little more cadaverous, the man downstairs – Dorian Grey – stays young, unbelievably young.

The notion of being able to stop the process of ageing – and halt the inevitable decline towards death – occupies us all at some time. Of course, death is unavoidable, but there needn't be anything foregone about the way we age. Thanks to amino acids we now have the power to slow down the ageing process. Amino acid therapy refutes the traditional, deeply-ingrained view that low energy and mental sluggishness, joint pains, loosening skin and constant infection are the unavoidable results of ageing. With the proper nutritional support you can, quite simply, live a longer, fuller and more vital life.

What is ageing?

One patient in his mid-fifties receiving nutritional counselling for arthritis described to us his feelings about ageing: 'To me getting old is like finding yourself in a prison. You gradually realize that things you had taken for granted – like a good, strong body and the ability to think clearly – were actually only special privileges that have now been withdrawn.'

To this man getting older was an unbearably frustrating experience. It prevented him from being as active as he once was and caused the levels of adaptive energy – the energy that allows us to respond to stresses with vigour – in his body to decline. Work became harder and the mental effort to get things done greater. His concentration started to slip and his memory falter. Sexual activity declined. He suffered from periods of apathy, depression and insomnia.

Perhaps the most common and harmful of all the consequences of growing old is that as a person ages his digestive system gets lazy. Stomach acid production slows down dramatically even by the age of forty. And by sixty almost one person in three secretes no acid at all. We've already seen how crucial the digestive system is to the body. Here in your gut the complex protein structures you eat are broken down into their simple building blocks – amino acids – before they are absorbed and reconstructed inside in the liver, pancreas and muscles as new and different protein structures. Think of this three-stage process – eating, digesting and rebuilding – as the swing of a pendulum. When we eat protein the pendulum is swinging upwards. When it is reconstructed it swings downwards. When the pendulum is frozen for a split second at its highest point, between the protein that was and the protein it will become, the food is in the digestion stage. Insufficient stomach acid simply arrests the downward swing causing a host of related health problems. When we lose stomach acid the enzyme-making pancreas is forced to secrete additional enzymes to compensate, from fewer available amino acids.

To cope with these additional demands the pancreas withdraws vitamins, minerals and aminos from other functions. These include arginine and ornithine, which are important for tissue repair and memory, histidine, which the body needs for adequate sexual response, and phenylalanine, which is necessary for stress support. In particular, many of the nutrients used in the immune system are diverted leaving the body vulnerable to the host of so-called age-related diseases such as arthritis, pneumonia and reduced resistance to infection.

Because of this, many nutritionists believe that supporting the body's digestive system with nutritional supplementation is a vital key in helping to keep you looking and feeling young. For example, one respected nutritional expert, D. Newbold, comments that he doesn't know of a single case of cancer, regardless of type, where the victim hadn't previously suffered from low stomach acid production. Not surprisingly the incidence of cancer rises dramatically with age.

The Demolition Men

As the immune system declines with a person's age (thanks in no small part to poor digestion), so does his resistance to toxicity from the environment. Heavy metals such as lead, cadmium and mercury are especially dangerous as they compete for absorption with beneficial trace elements such as zinc and selenium. A young, healthy body uses white blood cells (leucocytes) to repel these heavy metal invaders, but ageing leads to a decline in their numbers. When this happens the transport molecules used to carry zinc across the intestine mucosa – piccolinic acid – are effectively hijacked by the heavy metals. Zinc depletion is a major contributor to a loss of pliability in the skin and blood vessels as well as causing a decline in sperm production – all common symptoms of ageing.

Another problem with ageing is the action of free radicals. According to Pearson and Shaw in their book *Life Extension*, each quart of air contains a billion of these ravenous, destructive substances. Free radicals, as we have seen, are one of the main causes of allergies and indeed many illnesses, but when it comes to ageing they are particularly active. Let's see why.

In chapter 1 we explained how fibrous protein chains weave together into the strong, flexible cables of collagen. We then saw how collagen molecules mesh with each other like the branches of a hedge eventually forming tough, highly flexible organs such as skin, the heart, blood vessels, and so forth. If we were to look at these structures under a microscope the dense interlocking network of collagen cables would resemble a massive construction of builders' scaffolding. Now let's see what happens when a free radical forces its way into the structure. As long as it has its unpaired electron it possesses a positive charge, rather than the neutral charges of the molecules in the protein it has invaded. Therefore, to balance itself it naturally attracts charges from the surrounding molecules. But by robbing these charges from the collagen molecules it breaks open the peptide bonds and starts to dismantle the scaffolding-like molecules. This free radical activity causes a chain reaction as molecules from the broken chains – now ravenous for electrons themselves – try to rob other, neighbouring molecules of their electrons.

Now imagine a fraction of the billion or more free radicals contained in one breath of air, or caused by the ultra-violet rays of sunlight on your skin, affecting your body. When two free radicals meet, a cross-linkage of destruction occurs, undoing whole sections of scaffolding. In time the collagen molecules will collapse like a demolished tower block.

Of course, this destruction only takes place on a microscopic level and you won't suddenly find a pound of flesh falling off your arm (although free radicals are one of the causes of the dry flakiness of eczema). Instead, what you'll find is that your skin loses its softness and pliability and your face becomes gaunt, leathery and wrinkled. A good test for free radical activity is to pinch and lift the skin on the back of your hand then let it go. If it springs back into place the skin is healthy, but if it slow to return and retains a small, raised area where you pinched it then nutritional support is almost certainly called for. Of course, it's not just your skin that depends on collagen. Free radical activity damages capillaries as well, causing cardiovascular problems, restricting circulation and preventing nourishment from reaching the cells. Similarly, it can attack the alveoli of the lungs causing bronchitis and pneumonia. And it might alter DNA and RNA, leading to growths such as goitre and cancer.

Although free radical activity itself is one of the major causes of ageing, there are other factors which allow the free radicals to take hold. The decline of digestive functions with the resulting loss of enzyme production is a major cause. The body manufactures two particular enzymes to keep free radicals in check – superoxidase dismutase (SOD) and glutathione synthase. Children who suffer from a genetic disability to manufacture these two enzymes are victims of the illness progeria, where the unfettered free radicals cause them literally to grow old and die often before reaching adolescence. Supporting the pancreas with the materials it needs to create these anti-ageing enzymes has been shown to help victims of this awful disease. Many adults suffering from the same free radical damage are finding similar relief by taking the complete amino blend.

The Weight Dilemma

Another common cause of ageing is a decline in the work-rate of the endocrine organs. The most obvious symptoms of this are the loss of sexual appetite, decreasing growth hormone, fading levels of LH and FSH in women, and particularly a decline in the production of the immunity hormone, thymosin. Perhaps even more important is the way that thyroid gland activity slows down. As you age and the production of thyroxin declines the body needs fewer and fewer calories. Experts have estimated that after the age of twenty we need 1 per cent fewer calories each year. A person celebrating his seventieth birthday, therefore, needs only half the calories he would have wanted fifty years earlier. On the other hand his deteriorating physical state – poor digestion, reduced immunity – increases his body's need for the aminos, vitamins and minerals found in his food.

This dangerous nutritional dilemma faces everyone as they grow older. They can continue eating the same amount of calories to obtain the nutrition they need and in doing so risk heart disease, arterial sclerosis and obesity when the lack of thyroxin metabolizes their food inadequately. Or they can cut their calorie intake by eating less but starve their metabolic pathways of the nutrients they need for making protein structures such as tissue, enzymes and immune defences.

Before we go on to see exactly how aminos can help let's briefly sum up what we've seen so far: ageing is a process of degeneration caused by a complex co-relationship of factors. The slowing down of stomach acid production depletes the body's enzyme and immune systems. This leaves it open to attack from infection and free radical damage which hastens the ageing process. Much of the food which is eaten is used simply to support the beleaguered defences while tissue repair, sexual response and general vitality all decline. At the same time the slowing down of hormone production prevents what food remains from being metabolized effectively, leading to weight increase as well as further starving the body of essential nutrients.

These are some of the problems facing people as they age. Looking at the way each sympton of ageing contributes to the others it's hard to tell where and how the process really starts. Does acid and enzyme depletion lead to an increase in free radical activity or vice versa? No one is quite sure. What is certain is that ageing is a slow process, where recognizable symptoms gradually accumulate, and not some uncontrollable overnight metamorphosis. Hormone production declines gently; the same with acid and enzyme secretion. Therefore, if you anticipate and attack the deficiencies almost before they occur with properly chosen amino acids and associated nutrients you can stave off these symptoms. The skin's firmness can be prolonged and muscle tone retained; you can stay alert and active and free from disease much longer than you might ever have thought possible.

The Stay-Young Aminos

So what sort of programme should you follow? Remember that one of the most dangerous aspects of ageing is the decline in digestive functions. The enormous strain it places on the enzyme and immune systems lowers our resistance both to disease and the ageing effects of free radicals. We saw in the digestion chapter that one of the best ways to raise the levels of hydrochloric acid was with a dietary supplement of histidine, together with glutamic acid HCL, betaine HCL and glycine (see p. 92). We've also seen how important a complete blend of amino acids is in helping to relieve the stresses on the pancreas. It provides this most overworked of organs with additional amounts of all the raw materials it needs to fashion the protein-digesting proteolytic enzymes.

Although they are the very building blocks of your body, free-form amino acids are also very low in calories. Therefore, while the complete blend will help to replace the protein which is lost as you age, it will do so without causing an increase in weight. This helps to get around that awkward nutritional dilemma caused by thyroxin depletion. With our normal diets, which are relatively high in carbohydrates and cholesterol, we pay for the protein by having to take in fats and sugars at the same time. And while the endocrine system, particularly the thyroid gland, can metabolize this to release energy and promote muscle growth when we are younger, as we age these foods start to accumulate as fats. Taking much of the protein you need as free-form amino acids provides the necessary materials for maintaining muscle mass, replenishing worn-out protein in the organs and providing new enzymes and hormones, without the fear of putting on weight.

Cancer

One of the most horrific consequences of ageing is the increase in the incidence of cancer. If, as many experts believe, there is a direct relationship between low or non-existent stomach acid (and depleted enzyme levels) and cancer amino acids could prove invaluable. Already reports dating back to 1979 show that high doses of amino acids have been used successfully in cancer treatment. Cancer cells consume the amino acids in your body at a horribly fast rate. As the biochemist G. Guyton says: 'Cancer cells are prolific users of amino acids and, simultaneously, the proteins of other tissues become markedly depleted.' This means that when your resistance should be at its peak to fight the spread of cancer the nutrients your body wants to employ in making lymphocytes, interferon, antibodies, macrophages and enzymes are being swallowed by the tumour.

In a healthy body a shortage of the amino acids needed for a particular structure will force the body to dip into the circulating amino pools which is carried around in the bloodstream. To supply this pool the body might dismantle the protein chains of existing non-essential tissue to ensure that the supplies never become depleted. Cancer cells prevent this. Once an amino is absorbed into a cancer growth it becomes inextricably tied and contributes to the cancer's growth. As it grows it consumes more and more of the remaining amino-derived protein tissue. Meanwhile, in an attempt to combat the growing threat, the body sacrifices more of its own tissue to try and support the immune system – like having to rip up the proverbial floor boards to light a fire. Eventually, depleted both by the encroaching cancer and its own frantic self-destruction, the body dies. Nutritionists often refer to cancer as a protein-consumptive disease in which the victim is killed by a lack of protein. Protein is, after all, the most important substance in our bodies.

The great success of aminos in treating cancer stems – in addition to the way they improve digestion – from the fact that they can be given in very high doses to supplement the body's own depleted protein supply. Doses of the complete blend as well as individual aminos can be as high as 45 grammes a day. Some people argue that this feeds the cancer as much as it does the body, but their suggested alternative, of starving the body, hardly seems worth contemplating. Besides replenishing the body, the aminos can also be used to influence its anabolic/catabolic cycle. A cancer growth is after all only the anabolic phase gone haywire.

Anti-Ageing Chelators

So far we've seen how important the complete blend, together with the acid-generating aminos, is in combating ageing. Which other aminos should you take as part of a specific anti-ageing programme? Heavy metal toxicity poses such a threat to the body as it gets older that the chelating abilities of individual free-form aminos make powerful anti-ageing tools. The tripeptide amino glutathione – the combination of glycine, cysteine and glutamic acid – is looked upon by nutritionists as a 'chelator *par excellence*'. Experts find that it is effective in most cases of heavy metal poisoning and some factories in the USA are even giving it to their workers to protect them against high emissions of lead and mercury in the air. These metals are notorious for causing irritability and short-temperedness, and there are some tests to show that by oxidizing vitamin C they suppress the immune system. Glutathione works by transporting these harmful elements safely out of the body. Experts are currently using it to relieve nausea, hyperactivity and emphysema. Its chelating ability is also being used with great success to give help to arthritis sufferers.

Glutathione combines with the trace metal selenium to form one of the two natural free-radical-scavenging enzymes, glutathione synthase. We've seen how important this and superoxidase dismutase (SOD) are in stifling the chain reaction of ageing caused by free radicals. The immune system comes under a severe testing in later life and the support provided to it by glutathione make it one of the most important aminos you can take.

Histidine, as well as supporting stomach acid secretion and mediating your allergy response, is another excellent chelator. Besides glutathione and histidine there are several other aminos which, as we've seen in past chapters, also have a proven ability as chelators. They include methionine, cysteine and aspartic acid. Whether you choose to include them in a specific formula or prefer instead to take them as part of the complete blend is up to you.

Enervated Endocrines

While these aminos work as a shield against the ravages of poisoning and free radical damage, there are others you can take which will help to strengthen your body, raising it to an almost youthful level of efficiency. These are the aminos which supply and strengthen the endocrine organs, and regenerate fading hormone levels. We saw in chapter 13 how each of these aminos works. Arginine and ornithine stimulate the pituitary gland into releasing growth hormone (GH), which increases the muscle synthesis and mobilizes fat deposits. At the same time the amino tyrosine, together with co-factor iodine, raises the levels of thyroxin. When we are young we can eat platefuls of food, which is immediately burnt as energy or metabolized into muscle. This can happen because GH and thyroxin work synergistically to consume the food. Duplicating these youthful processes later in life by taking these three hormone-stimulating aminos is a method that many people, anxious to recover lost muscle tone have used with great success. In addition, the amino carnitine, together with vitamin C, helps to mount a lipotrophic – fat moblizing – rearguard action, scouring for arterial fat build-up and, in doing so, releasing more energy.

Arginine is also the precursor of spermine and spermidine. Chapter 4 showed us how these two chemicals relieve memory loss – surely one of the most confusing and disheartening aspects of ageing. They also work as inhibitory nerve chemicals, suppressing the tremors and motor tics which are another sign of the degeneration wrought by the ageing process. Another ageing illness associated with motor dysfunction is Parkinson's disease. Although there is no cure, many victims are prescribed doses of the catecholamine neurotransmitter L-dopa; so you may consider including the precursor phenylalanine, together with tyrosine. We saw earlier how another problem of ageing was a loss of adaptive energy, the simple inability to respond to stress, resulting in physical weakness as well as depression. In this case phenylalanine, as the precursor of noradrenalin and adrenalin, is a must.

Other beneficial aminos include tryptophan and GABA (Gamma Amino Butyric Acid) for their calming effects and taurine for its ability to transport calcium and sodium across the gut wall. Finally, cysteine is an amino which is becoming increasingly widely used to restore body to ageing hair. Of course, it's up to you which aminos you decide to include in an anti-ageing formula. Here as a guide are all the aminos we've mentioned in this chapter:

Aminos
histidine
betaine HCL
glycine
glutathione
arginine
ornithine
phenylalanine   (not to be taken with MAO inhibitors see p. 192)
tyrosine
GABA
cysteine
carnitine
taurine
Don't forget that supplements of the complete blend as a foundation to whichever aminos you choose will make an enormous difference.

Co-factors
A
B3
B6
B12
C
E
zinc
magnesium
selenium
calcium

Chapter 16

Youthful Skin Connection

Skin is the single biggest organ of your body. Like any other organ it plays a crucial role in the living process. It helps to regulate body temperature and is an important part of the immune defences, guarding against viral, fungal and bacterial infection. In this chapter we'll focus on ways of using amino acids to keep your skin soft, moist, pliable and looking young. Although the formulations we suggest you take are excellent for helping ageing skin, they can be used by anyone with skin problems – such as stretch marks or dry skin – or simply by those wanting protection from threats to their skin's health, such as ultra-violet light and pollution. We all need good skin, not just models and actors, and using free-form amino acids helps to ensure that's what we have.

Amino Sun-Spots

A hundred years ago porcelain-white skin was thought to be one of the greatest assets of a beautiful woman. Today the darker the tan you bring back with you from your holiday, the better. Although we find lustrous bronzed skin attactive, the damage which the sun's rays cause can often far outweight the benefits.

One of the most important factors in keeping your skin young-looking is the amount of moisture it retains. This is regulated by the prostoglandins, the chemicals derived from the unsaturated fatty acid, linoleic acid. Prostoglandins have many roles in the body. They play a part in immune response and lubricate connective tissue. They also account for the natural oiliness of our skin. This oiliness works to retain billions of water molecules in the tissue, keeping it well irrigated. When you lie on a blazing golden beach, no matter what factor of protective moisturized or sun-tan oil you apply, the sun's ultra-violet rays will penetrate the skin and start to oxidize these water molecules. This process robs water molecules of their electrons and in doing so it turns them into hydroxyls – the most dangerous of all free radicals. When hydroxyl production reaches a certain level it causes skin cancer. The destructive effect of ultra-violet light is one of the main reasons for the scientific world's current concern over the loss of the ozone layer from earth's upper atmosphere. The ozone layer filters out most of the ultra-violet that comes from the sun, effectively protecting us from a hydroxyl-induced cancer epidemic. For without this layer – and there is already a hole in it the size of Antartica caused by pollutants – skin cancer incidence would rocket.

However, even though most of the ultra-violet rays are screened and the levels of hydroxyl production in skin are generally low, sun-bathing still works to block the manufacture of prostoglandins from their fatty acid precursors. Without its natural moisturizer the skin can dry out very quickly. The best evidence of this is to be found on the beachside boulevards of such resorts as the Riviera and Los Angeles. The combination of smog and near-incessant sunshine has aged the skin of many sun-worshippers by ten or twenty years. Their skin looks leathery and wrinkled.

The safest protection against this damage is to sit inside during the fine weather and cultivate a delicate Victorian paleness. Alternatively, you can use amino acids and their co-factors to provide you with some really effective hydroxyl protection. We saw in the last chapter how successful glutathione is as a free radical scavenger. Taken together with the anti-oxidant vitamins A and C, glutathione can protect the prostoglandins and the stage-by-stage conversion which leads from linoleic acid. As heavy metals are another common cause of skin damage the chelating ability of glutathione should make it a compulsory part of every southern Californian's diet. Wherever you sun-bathe, though, whether it's at Biarritz or Blackpool, it's well worth including glutathione in your diet. As an alternative you might prefer to use each of glutathione's cheaper constituent aminos, glutamic acid, cysteine and glycine.

Sulphur-Based Skin Support

Staying in California for a moment, there are days in Los Angeles when the smog becomes so dense that, with the sun shining bleakly through, it casts an orange-yellow sheen on everything. This is due to the high levels of sulphur in the smog which is emitted in car exhaust fumes. Sulphur is one of the natural by-products of burning fossil fuels. The effects that power station emissions – high in sulphur – are having on the rivers, lakes and forests of Scandinavia and Germany is currently the subject of a major political controversy in Europe. One scientific conference was told recently how the sulphur, raining on the Black Forest in Bavaria as sulphuric acid, has already destroyed one tree in four. This is ironic because, as far as your skin is concerned, the revitalizing powers of sulphur are second to none. It protects against radiation, oxidation, heavy metals and hydroxyls and has been recognized for centuries as one of the best possible substances that you can take to give new life to tired skin.

Foods which are especially high in this remarkable mineral include garlic, onions and eggs. Supplements of the sulphur-based aminos, methionine, cysteine and taurine, will provide sulphur in some of its most concentrated and easily assimilated forms. Of these three aminos, experts find that cysteine is the most effective in relieving skin problems. This isn't surprising as a quarter of all the amino acids contained in collagen – the skin protein – are cysteine molecules. Without them collagen would simply fall apart. This is because cysteine's sulphur atoms link with each other in the spiral collagen helixes to form strong, flexible bonds, and these bonds help to maintain the helix structure. If you were to compare a collagen helix with the sort of spiral staircase that you sometimes see outside multi-storied buildings – their shapes are very similar – then each step of that staircase would be a cysteine bond, keeping the spiral shape intact. The free-radical-generated oxidation process that causes the skin to age works by undoing these bonds, making the spiral fall apart.

By ensuring that the body has supplemental cysteine if it needs it – in effect by flooding your metabolism with it – we can actually quench the free radicals' craving for the electrons in these bonds and prevent them from damaging the skin. Indeed, nutritionists often refer to cysteine and glutathione as 'free radical quenchers' – a phrase which actually sums up their role more accurately than the commonly used 'scavenger'. The remaining two sulphur-based aminos, methionine and taurine, are also very good quenchers – although they don't serve the same indispensible role in collagen formation as cysteine. Because of it's anti-free radical action 250 mg of cysteine a day is widely used as an anti-wrinkling supplement.

Stretching a Point

The problem of stretch marks is usually associated with pregnancy, but in fact it affects many people beside expectant mothers. These scar-like ribbons of diaphanous skin are responsible for a great deal of embarrassment and self-consciousness, not to say anxiety. Graham, a musician in his early twenties, complained of stretch marks that he had acquired as a result of weight lifting. 'Every time I

146

did a really good, hard workout I could feel my skin literally tearing,' he said. Rolling up his sleeves he uncovered his upper arms, revealing what looked like tiny, broken strands of silver on his skin. Stretch marks occur when the skin hasn't the elasticity to expand. Although it might feel perfectly pliable to the touch, the rigidity occurs at the molecular level. It often signifies a dietary deficiency of many important nutrients, particularly tryptophan and zinc. Zinc is the most important trace element in collagen. It lends the skin pliability and strength and to protect against further stretch marks and many nutritionists recommend taking it as a supplement, along with tryptophan.

Why take these two together? Basically, tryptophan helps to ensure that zinc is carried through the gut wall into the bloodstream. When zinc is digested it possesses a positive electronic charge; the gut wall it has to pass is negatively charged. As opposites attract, zinc has difficulty escaping beyond the wall into the blood. Instead it combines with the negatively charged carrier molecule piccolinic acid – one of the metabolic 'taxis' that we looked at earlier – and is then able to pass. The precursor of zinc's carrier molecule is tryptophan; you can see how crucial healthy tryptophan levels are for zinc absorption and so for good skin.

As well as cysteine we also recommend glycine in a stretch mark prevention blend. There are, in fact, even more molecules of glycine in each collagen chain than there are of cysteine. Glycine is a tiny amino acid which works in the collagen chains like the springs in a car suspension, absorbing the stresses and allowing it to flex without damage. Glycine deficiency make the collagen very brittle and some experts believe that this lack of 'give' is what leads to the sudden rupture of a stretch mark. Glycine, cysteine, tryptophan and zinc (together with vitamin C, which is another vital component of collagen as well as a remarkable anti-oxidant) make an excellent anti-stretching blend. For proof you only have to look at Graham. Within a few weeks of starting on this formulation, taking it together with the complete blend, his skin had stopped tearing and the existing marks were starting to clear up.

Skin Healing

Another form of skin damage that you can use aminos to help heal are the minor cuts and bruises of everyday life. Any wound, no matter how small, depletes the levels of arginine from the circulating amino pool. The lower the level sinks, the longer a wound will take to heal – especially if arginine is diverted into other functions such as supporting the immune system. Judith, a graphic designer, told us what happened when she accidentally cut her hand with a blade while trimming some card. As soon as it happened she bathed the wound, bandaged it and expected it to heal. Unfortunately, soon after this she caught a virus infection from her boyfriend. With most of the available nutrients expending themselves fighting the virus, there was little left of the amino pool to help the wound. As a result, starved of the nutrients it needed for repair, the cut became livid, swollen and painful.

At first she took the antibiotics her doctor had given her, but when these only gave her a headache she came for nutritional counselling. Her hand by now had become so swollen that she was unable to bend her fingers. Her lymph nodes too were swollen showing that her immune system was under great stress. She was immediately given the complete amino blend to stimulate the enzymes, the T-cells and the B-cells of the body. In addition, she was given extra supplements of arginine, glycine and cysteine to help the wound on her hand to heal. Within a few days the swelling where she cut herself had disappeared and by the end of the following week the large red weal it left had also gone.

Vitiligo

Another skin problem that responds to dietary supplementation with the complete amino blend is vitiligo. This is a disease that mainly effects people of Afro-Caribbean and Indian origin, destroying the pigment in their skin. It leaves large and unsightly, often symmetrical, white areas and it is a source of intense distress and anxiety. Experts think that, by raising enzyme production in the body, the complete blend will help to stimulate those enzymes responsible for the metabolic pathways of pigmentation.

One of the molecules needed for the pigment melanin is phenylalanine, and nutritionists speculate that using it together with folic acid and the complete blend will halt the spread of vitiliglio. It may even help to replace the pigment that has been lost.

As you can see, amino acids help to relieve a variety of skin-related problems. As well as those we've looked at, the complete blend, along with arginine and cysteine, also work well for acne and boils. On the other hand, if you suffer from eczema the allergy combination, of histidine and glutathione will help to clear it. Cold sores respond excellently to lysine – you can apply it directly to the affected area as well as administering it orally.

Skin complaints are more public than most health problems.

Short of hiding away, a victim of acne, or eczema or loss of pigmentation can't prevent his problem from being noticed. Of course, many people with skin complaints are happily unaffected by the anxiety that this problem causes others. Even so, in spite of this healthy and positive attitude, no one should ever be content with poorly conditioned skin. We know well enough by now that any health problem, whether it's eczema or arteriosclerosis, is only the most obvious symptom of much wider metabolic imbalances throughout the body of which we might be unaware. In this respect, the approach you take for revitalizing damaged or ageing skin is no different from the way you view any other health disorder. Whether you use amino acids simply to protect your skin from ultra-violet light when you go sun-bathing or as part of an anti-wrinkling programme, they will work to support your body by treating it for what it is – a single organism composed of thousands of interrelated pathways.

Chapter 17

Amino First Aid

So far we've seen how amino acids can be used to supplement those metabolic pathways which, by gradually becoming blocked and unbalanced, cause mental, emotional and physical illness. To get to the root of these problems amino acids and their co-factors usually take some time to effect relief. It might take a few days; it might even take a few weeks or, if the illness is a serious one such as heart disease, a few months before the full benefits of the orthomolecular approach are felt through the entire body. Because of the delayed, cumulative effects of these supplements you probably wouldn't expect them to be used for cases which demanded immediate treatment. If so, you couldn't be more wrong. To show you what we mean let's have a look at the benefits of giving amino acids to help victims of accidents or injuries.

Prompt treatment – providing immediate emotional and physical support – is crucial in those first moments following a trauma such as a car accident, bereavement, mugging or even rape. The sort of help given will play a major role in determining how quickly a victim recovers.

Amino Shock Troops

Perhaps the most effective area of amino first-aid care is the way these miraculous powders can work to protect the body from shock. In fact, if your metabolic pathways are well supplied your body is probably equipped to resist shock altogether. However, if you are unlucky enough to be a shock victim there are blends you can take which will help to offset its worst effects. Before we see which they are let's first discover what is meant by shock.

Shock is a violent response to sudden stress, physical, mental or emotional. We've all experienced the conditions that lead to this stress at some time in our lives. As we saw in chapter 5, although the exact circumstances may vary, an individual's physical and psychological responses are very similar to anyone else's. For example, when a dog runs out into the road and you have to slam on the brakes for an emergency stop, the heart palpitations and sudden perspiration are symptoms of mild shock. It's the same if you catch a flap of the stair carpet with your toe and fall downstairs. Even the hair-raised reaction to a horror film is a form of shock. Each of these examples leaves you with a racing heart beat, a queasy feeling in your stomach and a sudden sense of weakness and shivering.

These unpleasant physical sensations are, of course, the results of your body's sympathetic – fight or flight – nervous system. The diversion of blood away from the gut to the heavy muscles causes the nauseous sensation in your stomach, and the pounding heart beat is in fact the effort of your body to provide those muscles with the oxygen they need to perform. Meanwhile, the level of beta wave activity in your brain rises dramatically. This increases your alertness, allowing you to decide on a quick and efficient reaction – you are literally prepared to fight, or take flight from, the circumstances which caused the stress. You are aware of, and responsive to, everything around you, sensitive to the slightest change and ready to respond. Don't forget that here we're not just talking about violent physical stress. Sexual arousal causes the same responses, as does the exhilaration of a roller-coaster ride. Whatever the cause, the response is so far outside the body's normal functions that it places quite a strain on its resources.

Usually this fight or flight reaction is short-lived enough, and sufficiently mild, to leave you with nothing but a sense of fatigue. You might feel 'emotionally drained', but nothing worse. Sometimes, though, people are plunged into situations where a much more extreme response is demanded, and this response may upset the sympathetic/parasympathetic balance altogether. Kathy, herself an orthomolecular nutritionist, described to us an accident in which she was involved. She was a passenger in a car which hit a patch of black ice on the road, skidded and rolled down an embankment. 'Looking back on it I realize how acutely aware I was of what was happening. I remember watching the grass and the horizon "revolve" in slow motion – not just as a blur; I swear I saw every blade of grass. I also remember noticing a cloud in the sky which resembled one in a print I have at home.' Kathy's acute, dreamlike awareness – as if her senses had suddenly been amplified – is a typical effect of the sympathetic nervous system. The mind becomes highly alert and active. In fact, this alertness functioned far beyond her conscious state. 'I wasn't aware of my body at all,' she continued. 'It's as if it took care of itself without any conscious help from me.' When Kathy tried to recall how she had clawed her way out of the overturned car her mind was a blank. This highlights another aspect of the shock-related stress response: Kathy's reasoning ability was subordinated to her instinct – the instinct for survival.

Luckily, being a nutritionist, her body was well supplied with all the nutrients necessary for supporting these stress demands and she experienced no shock afterwards. For many people caught in this sort of situation, though, the sudden, extreme physical reaction has more lasting effects. We saw in chapter 5 just how dangerous uncontrolled stress can be. It prevents digestion and protein synthesis, slows down enzyme production and impedes the immune system. It can also result in chronic mood disorders. This is exactly what happens to many victims of shock. The immediate results may be stupor, torpor and unresponsiveness or alternatively extreme anxiety, perhaps even hysteria. Later it may lead to widespread nutritional deficiencies in the body, which in turn can lead to illness, infection and degeneration. Shock kills.

As shock – the prolonged physical and mental agitation resulting from an unbalanced autonomic nervous system – is only an extreme form of stress, one of the most important aims of first aid must be to administer sound nutritional support, particularly in the form of amino acids. So which aminos should you use? As we've seen, the shock trauma is likely to cause imbalances and blockages throughout the metabolic pathway network. Doses of a complete amino blend should therefore be included as the first line of defence against its effects. The complete blend will protect against enzyme depletion and support the immune system.

One of the characteristics of shock is that it often wedges its victims firmly into a beta wave state of mind. Even when the stress has passed they continue to respond in an abnormally sensitive fashion – even minor stimuli might cause a tearful, unreasoning and sometimes hysterical reaction. Therefore a blend which will calm the victim, encouraging alpha wave activity at the expense of beta waves, is important for helping to guard against long-term stress damage. The amino anxiety formula – tryptophan, histidine, glycine and taurine – is ideal for calming the patient in this way.

Histidine promotes alpha wave activity and works to counteract the highly-strung state of alertness caused by the beta waves. Tryptophan will back up histidine's calming effects, reacting synergistically to allow the autonomic nervous system to regain its balance. Giving the shock victim further supplements of tryptophan on top of the amounts contained in the complete blend and anxiety formula might be a good idea because of the way it will help the victim to get to sleep.

In the longer term you'll want to guard against post-shock depression. Like any stress – good as well as bad – shock will leave you drained of the nutrients you need for an adequate response to further stresses. When we've been under pleasant stress, the loss of the stressor – perhaps the excitement of visiting an exotic country – leads to a sense of anti-climax and melancholy. The same is true for the after-effects of shock. After expending so much energy and so many essential nutrients in responding to the situation, first by engaging the sympathetic nervous system and then by enduring the prolonged stress-related depletion of shock, your body is not left with very much for the necessary responses to the simple, everyday things such as work, friends and even getting up in the morning. You might sink into depression. Every action will become an effort, and concentration will seem impossible. This might also be compounded by an anxiety neurosis – an abiding fear of whatever it was that caused the shock. So providing your body with the nutrients which help it to rise to the normal demands of life is important.

The most effective of these nutrients are the aminos phenylalanine and tyrosine, as precursors of the catecholamines, and the brain fuel, glutamine. You might even choose to follow either the complete 'stresswatch' or depression formulas (see pp. 49 and 58) for a while to ensure that the amounts of those nutrients in your body are raised back to their pre-trauma levels. As basic shock support, though, these are the nutrients we recommend, taken twice a day until you feel they are no longer needed:

Aminos
tryptophan*
histidine
glycine
taurine
phenylalanine*
tyrosine
glutamine
(*not to be taken if you also use MAO inhibitors see p. 192)

Co-factors
B3
B6
C

As well as providing emotional and mental support, amino supplements can also be used to help the victims of physical injury.

The trauma of injury and the demands it makes on the body's supply of aminos, vitamins and minerals leads to nutritional depletion as rapidly as psychological stress. We've seen before how the levels of arginine drop greatly in an area of damaged skin or muscle. Therefore, this is one of the first aminos that should be given to an injured patient. Arginine also supports the thymus gland. The thymus-generated immune response is crucial in preventing infection from entering through the injured skin. The sulphur-based aminos, particularly cysteine, together with taurine, will also aid skin repair.

If muscle damage has occurred then it's best to add supplements of the branched chain amino acids – leucine, isoleucine and valine – to the formula. Unlike most aminos which are synthesized into protein structures in the liver, these aminos circulate directly to the areas of muscle where they are required and are then added to the protein chains which make up muscle fibre. Any muscle injury depletes the available supplies of the branched chain amino group, so supplementation is recommended.

Some nutritionists also give the branched chain aminos, together with arginine, in its role as the stimulator of growth hormone, and tyrosine, the precursor of thyroxin, to the victims of broken limbs. When a limb is being set it will be encased in plaster perhaps for many months. Unfortunately, the muscle which surrounds it tends to atrophy through disuse. Because of this, even after the plaster is removed, the patient must often undergo a further, tedious period of recovery, exercising the limb to promote a full return of muscle tone. But now, thanks to amino supplementation, experts feel that this muscle atrophy may be slowed down, or even prevented.

Try a blend like this twice a day:

Aminos
arginine
methionine
cysteine
taurine
tyrosine
leucine
isoleucine
valine

Co-factors
A
B3

B6
B12
C
zinc
calcium

For the bone itself, the best supplement to take is a complete amino blend. Bone is made with a latticework of peptide 'scaffolding', into which is mounted calcium phosphate. The peptides depend on a host of enzymes and aminos for their manufacture and any depletion can easily slow down the healing process. If, for example, the patient hasn't received full nutritional support to guard against the shock of his injury then the bone may mend a lot more sluggishly compared to the bone of a patient who has.

Infection Protection

Most of the book has concerned itself with ways of using free-form aminos to help relieve a variety of health problems. However, thinking of these marvellous supplements merely as remedies for pre-existing disorders or injuries greatly underestimates their potential. By strengthening the body's immune defences amino acids can be used to stop many of today's most common illnesses from occurring in the first place – particularly infections.

When a virus first invades your body, long before symptoms of the infection actually appear, the immune system, led by its T-cell lymphocytes, swings into action. The body creates each variety of T-cell, its B-cell antibodies and leucocyctes by drawing from the pool of circulating amino acids. When the invading virus is relatively insignificant the immune system is able to deal with it easily by using the readily available supplies of amino acids and co-factors. The chances are that we won't even be aware of this minor infection.

Every now and then we come into contact with stronger, more virulent strains of viruses. This puts far greater demands upon the immune system. Accordingly, the response must be much stronger. Antibodies, lymphocytes, lymphokines and macrophages have to be produced in large numbers to overcome the virus. But often there simply isn't a deep enough pool of circulating aminos to provide this massive response immediately. It takes time for the body to marshal its resources, tearing apart non-essential tissue to furnish the necessary aminos. While it assembles its forces the virus is free to take hold. Consequently, we come down with an illness and have to endure a slow recovery period as the immune system only gradually gets to grips with the infection.

However, if when you first come into contact with the infectant you can raise the circulating levels of those amino acids needed for the immune response you will stand a far better chance of resisting illness. Free form amino acids encourage the immune system to provide an immediate response without resorting to a costly time delay. Of course, often you don't realize that you've been infected until you actually start showing the symptoms. But there are other occasions – during a well-publicized flu epidemic, for example – when, by taking the complete blend, you can strengthen your immune system to a point where it might be able successfully to repel the virus. Many people take the complete blend, and co-factors, every day of their lives for just this sort of protection. Of course, if you are unlucky enough to come down with an infection, the complete blend will also help to speed up your recovery period – especially if you recognize the symptoms in their early stages.

Toxicity Tamers

The phrase 'environmental toxicity' covers a lot of ground, but perhaps the area receiving most attention is the topical concern about radiation poisoning. The recent fears caused by Chernobyl and persisting doubts about the safety assurances of nuclear officials in the West have led more and more people to nutritional supplementation to protect themselves from radiation. For example, news reports told how quickly chemists' stocks of iodine disappeared after the Chernobyl reactor explosion. As one of the main components of thyroxin, it helps to guard against thyroid cancer (caused by irradiated iodine) by saturating the thyroid with unradiated iodine. In fact, there are many other supplements that we can take for protection: the amino free radical scavengers are particularly effective.

In chapters 15 and 16 we saw how free radicals contribute to ageing, degeneration and cancer. Radiation, even low-level, is a major cause of free radical activity. It oxidizes water in the skin to make dangerous hydroxyl molecules, which may eventually lead to skin cancer. The free radical scavengers methionine and cysteine, together with their co-factors vitamin B3, B6, and C, and zinc, magnesium and iodine, can help to avoid much of this damage.

In addition to radiation, the levels of 'conventional' pollution seem to grow each year. The heavy metals which billow into the atmosphere from factory chimneys and car exhausts prevent your body from absorbing many of the vital trace elements. We've seen how chelation therapy combats this, using aminos to get rid of damaging heavy metals by clamping on to them and making it easy for the body to remove them. These chelator aminos – methionine, cysteine and glutathione – also make excellent supplements in the event of a nearby factory fire or if you have to work in an environment high in heavy metal toxicity.

As we've seen, it's almost impossible to impose boundaries on the health-enhancing potential of amino acids. Admittedly, when you give first aid treatment to a victim it's tempting to concentrate solely on the symptoms or the immediate effects of shock or injury and ignore the longer-term consequences. Very often, though, the seeds of further illness and degeneration are sown because of this attitude. That is, of course, unless full and adequate nutritional supplementation is provided as a component of the overall first-aid programme. With these nutrients you can ward off the emotional and psychological disorders of shock, support the body against any deficiencies that may result, and help to speed up wound-healing.

PART FOUR

CONFRONTATION WITH COMPULSION

Chapter 18

Kick Cigarettes with Amino Acids

The scene is a crowded north African night club. A pianist sings a plaintive lament to lost love. At his side sits a beautiful woman who gazes wistfully into space. The owner of the night club enters and, seeing the woman, his eyes narrow in a mixture of pain and wryness. Half mumbling, he utters one of the most famous lines of the century: 'Of all the gin joints in all the towns in all the world she has to come into mine.'

'Casablanca' is one of the world's great films. It is also arguably one of the most subversive. Next time you watch it see how the ever-present use of cigarettes is employed as a vital dramatic component. There is a great emotive charge in watching Bogart nonchalently light up (his face chiselled in highlight and shadow by the match flame), caught as he is between his love for Bergman and the danger of the Nazis. The rest of his world may be coming apart, but at least he can fall back for stability on his Marlboro'. His smoking seems to make his situation at once more realistic and more romantic. Yet today smoking is one of the world's biggest killers. Anyone who thinks it enhances their image or, worse, that it gives them physical or emotional support is living in a 'Casablanca' dream world.

Amino acids can't miraculously make you stop smoking. You must really want to do that yourself. If you do you will find them an invaluable aid in helping to ease the cravings which will follow. And more, they will give your body the nutritional support it needs to recover from the damage that smoking causes – improving your digestion, circulation and concentration and generally revitalizing your life.

The Killer Alight

If you smoke you are one of nearly twenty million people in Britain, or eighty million in the USA. Of this number 80 per cent of men, 60 per cent of women, consume at least one packet a day, despite the overwhelming evidence that shows it causes lung, stomach and bladder cancer, bronchitis and influenza, ulcers and heart disease. If

161

you smoke heavily the cholesterol levels in your blood may be six times as great as those of non-smokers. In other words, there is a good chance that large fat deposits are forming in your blood now, making your arteries harden and raising your blood pressure. Normally our bodies are full of biochemical checks and balances to stop this from happening. Zinc, for example, is used by the body to keep arteries in good condition. But cadmium, a heavy metal found in cigarette smoke, displaces zinc. The lungs also need zinc to maintain their elasticity, which is why so many smokers, their lung tissue starved of zinc, suffer from emphysema.

Smoking causes an excess in your blood of another natural opponent of zinc – copper. A small amount of copper is needed for haemoglobin, the oxygen-carrying blood cells. But larger amounts oxidize vitamin C. Among its many duties, vitamin C is responsible for the upkeep of blood vessels, cleaning out the cholesterol and maintaining the fibrous collagen. Vitamin C deficiency (and 25 mg are destroyed with each cigarette) raises blood pressure – leading to heart attacks and strokes – and makes your skin age prematurely.

Excess copper also creates the enzyme histaminase, which breaks down the highly active amino, histamine. Without enough histamine your body won't produce sufficient stomach acid to digest your food properly. Your immune system will succumb to infection more easily. As well as losing your sex drive, you might fall prey to anxiety and schizophrenia.

The reaction that occurs between another metal in the tobacco, nickel, and the carbon monoxide, which is released when your cigarette burns, produces nickel carbonyl – a lethal oxidizing agent. Carbon monoxide on its own combines with the oxygen-carrying haemoglobin to produce carboxy haemoglobin. This stable compound is what makes the exhaust fumes in your garage so dangerous. It destroys brain cells by starving them of oxygen.

Nicotine also interferes with the release of hormones. By raising insulin secretion from the pancreas it robs the brain of its major fuel, glucose (the other being the amino, glutamine). This often causes fatigue and dizzy spells and may even result in hypoglycemia. Nicotine also causes up to an 80 per cent increase in blood adrenalin levels. At first this might make you anxious and nervy. Later as the adrenalin levels begin to drop it will exhaust you and might even lead to chronic depression.

The degeneration that smoking causes accumulates slowly in the body. So slowly that you might not notice the loss of taste in your food, the poor digestion, your developing night-blindness, the short temper, the anxiety, even the difficulty you have breathing. Not notice, that is, until you stop smoking and realize the difference.

If you smoke you probably get tired of pious non-smokers lecturing you about giving up. You might have your own reasons for smoking which they refuse to understand. Even if you do want to stop these reasons will play heavily on your mind. So before we look at how to give up let's examine the arguments you might give for carrying on smoking.

Smoking Reasons

One reason for smoking – particularly when you start and the novelty is fresh – is the thought that it enhances your appearance. Does it? Recently we watched a ten-year-old playing football in a playground. Every so often he took a drag from the cigarette he held between his thumb and forefinger, closing his eyes each time as if in rapture. He was acting the role of the nonchalent male and must have thought he looked marvellous. What he looked was absurd. No one needs to act a part at all and to do it by polluting your body is tragic.

Smoking also allows you to waste time. You might take a drag on your cigarette before answering a question. It gives you time to gather your thoughts. Then there is the tactile quality of your cigarette. It is something to hold on to, to fidget with. 'If I'm at a stand-up party,' said one smoker, 'I must have a drink in one hand and a cigarette in the other so I won't feel awkward.'

People also imagine that cigarettes relieve tension. They're wrong. What relaxes you is the stretching of your lungs as you take a drag rather than actually inhaling the tobacco. Watch people when they are tense or frightened; they gasp involuntarily to relieve their anxiety. In other words, you will get as much relief just from breathing deeply.

Last is the addiction. Your body quickly gears itself to the abnormal demands that smoking makes (such as increasing the blood adrenalin levels). Stopping suddenly disorientates the metabolism. You become nervous, drowsy, anxious; you suffer from loss of energy, sweating, cramps, tremors and palpitations. Put simply, you need a nicotine fix. Paradoxically, this is one of the factors that makes smoking so attractive. Because, unlike most areas of our lives it is a desire for satisfaction that you can easily meet. 'Simply by lighting up I'm achieving a little victory against adversity,' said a patient, 'So why should I stop?'

These reasons, the last especially, are what makes smoking such a difficult habit to give up. However, if you really do want to stop you can. Let's see how to cope with the physical and mental addiction. Then we'll examine the way the metabolic family of amino acids, minerals and vitamins can help you to stop smoking, quickly restoring your body's health and vitality.

Starting to Stop

Once you have decided that you want to give up don't get carried away. You must remember that when you first started you probably only smoked the odd cigarette now and then rather than the packet a day or more that you smoke now. Consequently, your physical and psychological dependence will have grown slowly, the destructive effects accumulating almost unnoticed. If you don't realize how nicotine-dominated your body is you will probably try to give up totally in one go. This is too drastic. It almost always leads to acute withdrawal symptoms as the body is suddenly deprived of nicotine. The anxiety and craving that result might well drive you straight back to the cellophane-wrapped packet.

Instead, what you should do is slowly and methodically cut cigarettes out from particular times of your day. Then, using the remarkable calming and strengthening powers of amino acids, prepare yourself to withstand the withdrawal symptoms when they happen. In this way you can control the cravings rather than allowing them to, control you.

First, think of all those activities which involve lighting a cigarette – speaking on the phone, for example, or travelling to work, or making a cup of tea. Pick one out and then stop yourself from ever lighting up in that situation again. Gradually widen the list of smoking-excluded activities so that finally there are only small pockets left in your day when you can smoke. Then, when you do smoke, take no more than three drags from the cigarette. This will satisfy your addiction without actually strengthening it.

No matter how slow this process is your body will start reacting to the physical changes. You might suffer from periods of fatigue or excess energy. Your head will start to ache and you will feel sick. You will probably start fretting and feeling sorry for yourself. The pressure to smoke will be intense, not helped by friends at work, smoky pubs and devious advertising hoardings. You will pass through phases of depression, resentment and anger. This is where amino acids really come into their own. By promoting a more tranquil and relaxed state of mind they will leave you much more able to cope with the anguish of withdrawal.

Helpers

Histidine is probably the most beneficial amino you can take to help you overcome your cravings. When you smoke the copper you breathe in as part of the cigarette smoke metabolizes in your body to create the enzyme histaminase. This in turn breaks down the histamine. As we have seen, histamine is an important neuro-inhibitor (Dr Carl Pfeiffer has found that when brain and blood levels of histamine were either high or low the patients suffered from over-stimulated and anxious behaviour). Histamine works in the brain by increasing the intensity of the relaxing alpha waves – and so reducing the stimulant beta waves. Taken as a supplement, histidine, histamine's precursor, helps to relieve your anxiety and fretfulness, leaving you more composed, relaxed and objective.

As the precursor of serotonin, the amino acid tryptophan makes another excellent dietary supplement when you stop smoking. Like histamine, serotonin deficiency can lead to anxiety, tension and depression. Research measuring the brain waves of volunteer patients shows that about forty-five minutes after taking trypto-phan, and it's conversion in the body to serotonin, their waking states become much more relaxed and tranquil. This helps you to decide which parts of the day you will stop smoking. You can take a tryptophan supplement in advance to ease the anxiety you feel when you stop. When you take tryptophan, you will probably find that it extends the periods you can go without cigarettes for much longer throughout the day. Unlike man-made tranquilizers, it won't interfere with your day's work by making you drowsy.

Smokers often find they are helped by taking the entire anxiety formula (see p. 66). Roger, a former heavy smoker, is the owner of a small builder's merchants. His stock yard is accessible only through a narrow alleyway and as there is no room to turn in the yard he has to reverse his lorry up the alley when he delivers or collects materials. It's a skilful, and physically demanding, manoeuvre, with only inches to spare on either side. He has to be alert and sensitive to the handling of the lorry.

'It annoyed me,' he said. 'Because once my lorry was in the yard the first thing I did was put a cigarette in my mouth. I realized that any pressure on me, like reversing in here, made me immediately light up. I'd been thinking of giving up for some time so I finally decided to give it a go. The trouble was that when I did give up I got short-tempered really easily, and I became forgetful and clumsy. When it came to reversing up that alley I was terrible. I just couldn't keep a straight line. I kept overcompensating with the steering-wheel so that I scraped first one wall then the other. When I reached

the yard my hands were shaking and I was gasping for a cigarette.'
Luckily, instead of giving in to the anxiety, the mental instability
and physical lack of coordination, he followed a friend's advice and
tried the amino anxiety formula. It did the trick. He hasn't smoked
since, and neither has his lorry scraped the alley walls.

Depression

As well as the sort of anxiety felt by Roger, many smokers have to
weather periods of torpor and depression when they give up. It's as
if without cigarettes they simply have no will or energy of their
own. The stress of giving up and the way it depletes the body of
essential nutrients may be one cause of this. Another is the
readjustment the body makes after having met the exceptional
demands of the nicotine for so long. Remember that nicotine can
cause massive increases in the circulating levels of adrenalin. This is
the end-product of the body's excitory stress pathway and continual
stimulation effectively turns you into an adrenalin junkie. So when
the levels begin to sink you will almost certainly feel depressed.
Without the natural nicotine stimulant you might find it hard to
respond to stress when you have to. Smokers often say that cigarettes
pick them up. The fact is that cigarettes create the depression in the
first place.

The aminos, phenylalanine and tyrosine, are the best supplements to take when you feel like this. They are the precursors of the
excitory catecholamine neurotransmitters and if they are depleted
you simply won't be able to respond to stress when it occurs. They
help to replenish circulating levels of noradrenalin and adrenalin,
both of which are vital in giving you the energy to respond to stress.
Methionine – taken with phenylalanine and tyrosine to help the
conversion of noradrenalin to adrenalin – is also a highly effective
aid in picking you up.

Sugar problems

Another cause of this depression may be connected with your
insulin levels. Insulin is the hormone produced in the pancreas
which regulates the amount of sugar that the body and brain
receives. Nicotine fools the body into thinking that there is more
sugar circulating than there really is. Insulin is then secreted to
lower these phantom blood sugar levels by encouraging the liver to
store the sugar as glycogen. In fact, as your sugar levels are probably
normal this storage process will dangerously reduce them. The

results can be dizziness, faintness, irritability, nervousness and, of course, depression.

Recently a French research team headed by D. Bacques found that blood sugar levels can be regulated by certain free-form amino acids. Bacques discovered that there is an equilibrium between phenylamine and the concentration in the body of glucose. He also found that the aminos glutame, glycine and lysine are hyperglycemic, which means that they raise blood sugar levels. They are now widely used to relieve low blood sugar, particularly from cases of post-smoking depression. Furthermore, as well as glucose, glutamic acid is a brain fuel in its own right. It heightens your alertness and allows you to think more clearly.

Getting Better

Unlike conventional drugs, amino acids work synergistically – taken to strengthen one metabolic pathway they help to strengthen many others. So when you take these aminos they won't just help you to fight the cravings, the anxiety, tension, fatigue and depression; they will also prove invaluable in helping your body to recover from the biochemical damage of smoking. Your digestion will improve. Food will taste so good you might think that up until now you had been wearing a sock over your tongue. Your improving physical wellbeing (at a drastically faster rate thanks to the amino acid supplements) will naturally add momentum to your desire to give up totally.

Histidine, for example, does so much more than simply help you to relax. It is also an excellent heavy metal chelator. The heavy metals in cigarette smoke – chromium, cadmium and copper – attack the body like mindless vandals in a football crowd. They oxidize vitamin C (leading to poorly formed collagen, restricted blood vessels and premature ageing), form enzymes which break down amino acids and antagonize other minerals like zinc (which is needed everywhere in the body, from the lungs to the prostate gland). Happily, both histidine and histamine render these heavy metals harmless by chelating them out of the body. Histamine will also help to improve your digestion by increasing the secretion of stomach acid.

Cigarettes and Weight Gain

For many ex-smoker's one of the most distressing results of stopping is finding that without cigarettes they tend to put on weight very quickly. There are several reasons for this. For instance, the stress that giving up causes elicits a response from the sympathetic nervous system. One way to counter this is to eat more. Many people, without realizing it, eat when they are anxious, whether it is about failing their driving test or giving up smoking.

Others use eating as a substitute for the time-wasting that they used to get away with by smoking. When you stop you suddenly find yourself with a lot of spare time and it must be tempting to fill it by eating an extra snack or two. Furthermore, with your digestion improving as a result of giving up smoking you will probably feel hungrier. You might have to eat more at mealtimes just to feel sated.

These factors tend to act upon each other, making the weight gain sometimes very dramatic. To prevent this from happening many nutritionists have found phenylalanine to be a marvellous appetite suppressant. Research shows that it triggers the release in the gut of the neurotransmitter-type substance cholycystokinin (CCK). Normally this chemical is secreted when food levels in the stomach are high to tell the brain that the body has eaten enough. The hypothalamus then registers a feeling of satiety. Giving phenylalanine to raise CCK levels will give you the same feeling without having to overeat. Taken at bedtime phenylalanine can help to reduce your cravings for sweets and snacks between meals.

Carnitine is another amino that helps to prevent weight gain. It is used to stimulate fat metabolism in patients suffering from obesity. The fatty acids can then be transported across the cell membranes into the mitochrondria, where they are burnt as energy sources.

When all is said and done, the hardest thing about giving up is to convince yourself that you need to. Every fact, every awful detail about the havoc it wreaks in your body won't make the slightest difference unless you truly want to stop. If you do make the decision you can depend on amino acids to help you overcome the enormous hurdle of the physical and mental cravings. What's more, they will be there to catch you as you come down on the other side – renewing your body's vitality, proving that your decision to quit was the right one.

Chapter 19

Aminos Against Alcoholism

'It's been awful. He was sacked from his job about four months ago because of his drinking. He's in his late forties and his boss refuses to give him a reference, so even if he does come off the bottle he's virtually unemployable. We've had to sell the house and we're up to our neck in debt. I'm working as a waitress in a coffee shop. It's the only income we've got coming in. He's no help at all. The other day he said: "I'm just popping out to buy a paper," as charmingly and breezily as possible. Three hours later I got a call from a pub owner asking me to come and collect my husband. He was leaning against the bar dead drunk and when he saw me come in he said: "Oh, here she is. Madam high and mighty. Why don't you leave me alone." This was in front of a bar full of regulars. He just doesn't realize how cruel he is. If I try to stop him from drinking or reason with him he says that I don't love him anymore. I don't think he really believes he has a problem at all which is why he can't understand why I get so angry. He's never hit me but the way I've been abused and degraded is ... is ... He just doesn't consider my feelings at all. It's hopeless. I'd leave him but where can I go?'

Alcoholism is the fourth largest illness in the world, beaten only by heart disease, cancer and mental illness. It shortens the average lifespan by eleven years. For every healthy person who decides to commit suidice there are sixty alcoholics. Putting aside for a moment the emotional traumas that it causes, the physical ravages alone are appalling – inflammation and scarring (cirrhosis) of the liver, loss of memory, widespread haemorrhaging and obesity. Not to mention the defects in babies born to alcoholic mothers – the deformed limbs, distorted faces and weak hearts.

The opening paragraph of this chapter is a quote from a woman called Deborah. She brought her husband, Geoff, to nutritional counselling in a last bid to save their marriage – and possibly his life. Geoff's decline into alcoholism had followed the classic progression of minute, almost unnoticed stages. He had always enjoyed drinking socially. One reason, he later confessed, was due to his unease in company – a few drinks relaxed him, allowed him to become friendly and expansive and he liked thinking of himself as the outgoing centre of attention. Gradually, though, he started to drink for the sake of drinking. At work he spent most lunch hours at the pub, usually on his own; at home he got through three bottles of gin a week. If Deborah asked him not to drink so much he'd use the opportunity to start an argument. It always ended in him angrily walking out of the house. What he refused to admit at the time was that he caused the argument to justify having to go to the pub to 'cool off'.

At work Geoff began to suffer from lapses of memory – forgetting the names of clients, colleagues and, occasionally, even his secretary. When he found himself under pressure he would experience an immediate loss of confidence, start to panic and find it impossible to stop his hands from shaking – at least, without a drink. He realized later how obvious his drinking must have seemed to his colleagues but at the time he thought he had everything under wraps. 'Once in the lift someone jokingly warned against putting a match near my mouth for fear of blowing the building up,' he recalled. 'Well I turned on him, shouting and ranting, saying that if he had something to say he should say it and telling him to mind his own business both at the same time.'

He was now drinking continually. He started blacking out and suffering for days on end from nausea and fatigue. He had lost thirty pounds. The flesh on his face sagged and the tiny cheek capillaries haemorrhaged, giving him a haggard, bruised appearance. He urinated frequently, and painfully. His joints ached and the small of his back felt like a punch bag. Finally, on the recommendation of his doctor he was admitted to a hospital specializing in alcoholic rehabilitation. In addition to the group therapy and the classes on the damage that alcohol causes, he was made to take Metronidozole. This drug causes violent physical reactions such as stomach cramps, convulsions and nausea whenever the victim drinks spirits. A strong aversion to alcohol is meant to result. Within a month of leaving hospital, Geoff was drinking again.

Finally, on the advice of a friend, Deborah brought Geoff to nutritional counselling. They were shown how amino-based nutritional therapy attacks alcoholism from a radically different angle to conventional treatments. Nutritional counselling looks wholly to inadequate nutrition as the root of the problem rather than outside events that might be said to have 'driven him to drink'. Instead of using normal rehabilitative programmes which employ pain, stress and emotional pressure to force the alcoholic to give up, amino therapy involves locating the damaged metabolic pathways, those affecting emotional behaviour as well as physical well-being, then supplementing and 'repairing' them with an effective blend of amino acids.

Three months after his first consultation Geoff was a new man. He had stopped drinking completely and his marriage was on the mend. He had also received the offer of a job from a newly-established engineering firm. Each amino constituent of the formulation used to help Geoff was included for the unique way it helped to fight his alcoholism. We'll look at each of these aminos one by one and then examine the formula Geoff used at the end of the chapter.

Sucrose Staunchers

The first thing to do when treating an alcoholic is to try and stop him from wanting to drink. For this reason the first amino we'll look at is glutamine. It is simply one of the most effective supplements available for relieving the alcohol craving. It works very differently from the drugs that Geoff was given in hospital. Those drugs lead to the sort of violent, extremely painful reactions which are meant to drive an alcoholic to develop an aversion to alcohol. The theory is that the patient, equating his sudden nausea and wrenching stomach cramp with the drink, becomes conditioned to stop drinking. In many cases, however, no sooner have the effects of the drug worn off than the victim's craving returns. Glutamine, on the other hand, is successful because, rather than bullying the alcoholic into stopping, it gently suppresses the mechanism in the brain which causes his craving. It eradicates the compulsion to drink which is often such an obstacle to giving up.

Experts think that it does this by working on the appetite centre of the brain's hypothalamus gland. The appetite centre's function is to interpret how little or how much food there is in the body. If, for example, you haven't eaten for some time and your body is short of nutrition, the appetite centre will secrete hormones which make you feel hungry. Or, more specifically, if your body is short of a particular food, the appetite centre creates a craving for that one food. When you indulge the craving, by eating the food in excess, the nutritional balance is restored.

In the case of alcoholism, many of the people driven to excessive drinking suffer from extremely low blood sugar (hypoglycemia). Responding to this, the appetite centre creates an urge to consume foods that raise the levels of sugar circulating in the blood – an urge which, as far as the body is concerned, alcohol meets very successfully. The drawback to this is that, despite the way that alcohol initially increases the amount of blood sugar, in the longer term it actually causes a drop in these sugar levels. To compensate the appetite centre increases the desire for sugar; the alcoholic drinks more, causing the levels to drop even further, and so on.

But why should the body want to create a craving for alcohol if it causes the sugar levels to fall? This initial rise (and subsequent fall) in sugar levels caused by alcohol occurs because of the type of sugar which alcohol contains. Known as sucrose, it has almost no energy value at all. A term commonly used to describe it refers to its 'empty calories'. Unfortunately, our bodies have no mechanism to distinguish between this sugar and the other, nutritious form glucose. So when sucrose circulates in the blood the body perceives it as the useful glucose and secretes insulin to store it. It is collected and stored in the pancreas.

Unlike glucose, which is a brain fuel, sucrose is nutritionally useless. It serves no purpose in the body at all other than causing glucose depletion. The results of this depletion will include fatigue, sluggish reactions, reduced awareness, sleepiness and depression. All these disorders are recognized by the brain as symptoms of low blood sugar levels. To restore blood sugar it orders the appetite centre to create a sugar craving. Unfortunately, this only serves to increase the victim's alcohol craving.

Glutamine can break this vicious circle wide open. Remember, glutamine suppresses the brain messages which cause the sugar craving. This allows the blood sugar levels gradually to return to normal and eradicates one of the main reasons for an alcoholic's inability to stop drinking. As it works for any sort of carbohydrate fixation and not merely alcohol, glutamine also helps to improve a patient's general eating habits. Alcoholics notoriously choose foods with a high carbohydrate content which, as well as strengthening the alcohol addiction, also leads to digestive problems, obesity and heart disease. Glutamine, therefore, is indispensible for the treatment of a variety of alcohol-related disorders.

Glycine is an amino acid which is often used with glutamine to help relieve the hypoglycemia and cravings of alcoholism. It stimulates the release of glucagon from the pancreas. This is one of the body's own sugar-regulating molecules and it helps to raise sugar levels to normal.

Leaving Leucine Alone

However, amino acids aren't always so beneficial. For example, excess amounts of the amino leucine provide another contributiing factor in lower blood sugar levels. Nutritionists have found that alcoholism actually increases the levels of leucine in the body and this is likely to contribute to the victim's hypoglycemia. More importantly, excess leucine can wreak a variety of mood disorders and physical complaints which only make it harder for the alcoholic to stop drinking. These are caused because leucine makes the kidneys spill niacin wastefully into the urine. Niacin (vitamin B3) is an essential component in thousands of metabolic pathways. It assists in the breakdown and utilization of fat, protein and carbohydrate. It helps give pliability to the capillaries and is used in the immune response. Niacin deficiency is a cause of the disease pellagra – its symptoms are weakness, diarrhoea, dermatitis and nervous mental disorders like psychosis and anxiety. Niacin also regulates blood sugar levels, helping to avoid hypoglycemia. Niacin deficiency is one of the reasons why alcoholism so closely resembles schizophrenia: the abnormal use of carbohydrate and the mental and emotional disturbances are common to both diseases.

Niacin is just too important to do without altogether. So, when leucine causes a niacin deficiency the body turns for help to the amino acid, tryptophan. As we've seen before, one of trytophan's metabolic pathways produces nicotinic acid, a form of vitamin B3. Unfortunately, as it takes 60 mg of tryptophan to create 1 mg of B3 this in turn creates a dangerous tryptophan deficiency. Tests conducted on the urine of chronically alcoholic patients show, for example, that production of the inhibitory neurotransmitter serotonin suffers a drop of 40 per cent in the body. This drop is probably another reason for the mood disorders experienced by alcoholics. We've seen repeatedly how tryptophan, by way of its serotonin-producing pathway, works to relieve stress, anxiety and depression. Insufficient serotonin prevents you from sleeping soundly and can even lead to aggression and unreasoning anger. All of these symptoms are typical of chronic alcoholism, and are all caused in a roundabout way by the excess leucine.

In time, other processes begin to suffer too. Zinc, for instance, is prevented from being absorbed from the gut by a lack of tryptophan. How does this happen? Simply because no substance which is digested in the gut can pass through the intestine wall without a carrier molecule. When the structure of one of these molecules matches those of particular digested chemicals, it picks them up and shuttles them through the gut wall like a metabolic taxi.

The taxi which zinc needs for its journey is the tryptophan-derived piccolinic acid. No tryptophan, no taxi. Much of the zinc simply sits in the gut doing nothing until it's excreted. Zinc is needed everywhere in the body, for elasticity of lungs and capillaries, for bone structure, enzyme production and fertility. Many of the phsyical disabilities of alcoholism such as stiffness, haemorrhaging of skin capillaries and impotence can be attributed to zinc deficiency.

All these problems can be traced back to excess leucine. Reducing the levels of this amino is therefore an ideal way of helping to rehabilitate an alcoholic – raising blood sugar levels, dispelling emotional disorders and encouraging greater physical well-being. How do you go about reducing leucine? First, you have to realize that as well as isoleucine and valine, leucine is a branched chain amino acid (BCAA). This means that all three must share identically structured transport molecules across the intestine wall.

To illustrate this point think of the BCAAs in the gut – released from the protein chains and individually waiting for absorption – as a queue of travellers standing at a taxi rank. As there are fewer taxis than people, many travellers will have to wait before they can get a ride. In the same way, the branched chain aminos virtually have to queue up to be transported in the bloodstream. Therefore, raising the levels of one of these aminos – by taking it as a supplement – will lead to a depletion of the other two by hogging more of the available transport molecules. Therefore, by taking supplements of isoleucine, one of the competing BCAAs, you can actually reduce and regulate the amount of leucine which is absorbed.

In addition to the isoleucine, you can also take supplements of tryptophan, vitamin B3 and zinc. This will have the effect of strengthening each of the metabolic pathways that radiate out from tryptophan like the spokes of a cart-wheel. Zinc increases the well-being of tissue; B3 supplements will save having to use up excessive amounts of tryptophan to make nicotinic acid; and serotonin will work to relieve the alcoholic's anxiety and melancholia.

Cell Support

A lot of the recent research conducted into how and why alcohol affects mood has centred on the way it disrupts the function of brain cells (neurons). Like all cells, the surface membranes of neurons are made of a double skin of fat compounds. Piercing these fatty membranes, jutting out from the cell as well as penetrating them, are many thousands of protein structures which act as receptor sites. These sites are responsible for secreting the neurotransmitting chemicals which convey brain messages across the space between each cell. The uninterrupted passage of impulses along the entire nervous system depends on the efficiency of these receptor sites.

One of the factors which ensures this efficiency is that the fatty cell membranes in which the receptors sit are slightly fluid. This fluidity allows the receptors to move around on the surface. The importance of this mobility is that it allows the receptor sites to align themselves very precisely. They can direct themselves like antennae. This direction finding ability is important because in order for a specific brain message to pass from one cell to the next the structure passing the message on has to locate the similar receptor on the next cell which is designed to receive it.

To put it another way, the thousands of different receptors speak thousands of different languages – one for every sort of message. When a receptor which speaks one language passes a message on it can only be received by another which speaks the same language. So the slightly fluid surface of the cell lets the receptors quickly and efficiently reposition themselves when searching for another receptor of the same 'language'.

Alcohol, however, disrupts this process. This is because it is a solvent. The cell wall reacts to it by becoming more fluid – like treacle turning to water – and the balance between mobility and rigidity is tipped over. With nothing to coordinate their messages the receptors are sent haywire – firing off their neurotransmitters without properly aligning themselves so that their messages are received by receptors which speak different languages.

Not surprisingly the brain messages become scrambled. Motor commands from the brain to your limbs are garbled, resulting in the loss of balance and coordination typical of drunkenness. Speech centres are affected (you only have to listen to a drunk person talking – his speech is so slurred that his tongue sounds as if it is hamstrung). Contrary to popular belief, it is much harder to get to sleep if you are drunk. Particularly interesting is the way that the receptors which convey pain messages are knocked out. This accounts for the opiate-like feeling of elation that alcohol gives. It also leads to an excess of the excitable neurotransmitter noradrenalin. This is why many people become noisy, agitated and aggressive when they drink.

Slowly, however, the membranes begin to adapt to the effects of alcohol. To do so they absorb greater amounts of cholesterol and mineral-based fat compounds. This has the effect of making the cell walls very much more rigid. It also accounts for the alcohol tolerance which develops as ever greater quantities of alcohol are needed to make the cell walls reach that state of fluidity which causes drunkenness. The alcoholic is constantly increasing his consumption of alcohol simply to reach the same state of euphoria. The resulting depletion of blood sugar only serves to make him drink more. As we've seen with Geoff, the process quickly spirals out of control.

It also makes it immensely difficult for a chronic alcoholic to stop drinking. By this time the only way he keeps the walls of his brain cells in an even normal state of fluidity is by drinking excessively. In Malcolm Lowry's extraordinary book about an alcoholic, *Under the Volcano*, the drunken hero, Geoffrey Firmin, recognizes 'this precarious stage, so arduous to maintain, of being drunk in which he alone was sobre'. If the alcoholic stops drinking he is depriving the cell walls of the solvent to dilute them, yet by this time they have adapted themselves to absorb much more hardening material than normal. As a result they become very rigid.

This rigidity also causes major problems. First it leads to a depletion of neurotransmitters – particularly noradrenalin. As we saw in chapter 6, noradrenalin deficiency is a major cause of chronic depression. It leads to fatigue and torpor, a general lack of interest in life which, if allowed, soon leads to physical and mental illness. Second, the alcoholic experiences confusion and pain, sometimes even blackouts, as the neurotransmitters which are produced fail to connect with the correct receptors on the now immobile surfaces of the cells. The anxiety, drop in body temperature and acute shivering of delerium tremens are common results of this.

In these conditions how could an alcoholic possibly stop drinking? The answer is by using amino acid supplements. Admittedly, the trauma that giving up causes is intense, but by using amino acids to support the body as alcohol is withdrawn many of the symptoms can be avoided altogether. To combat the mental fatigue caused by noradrenalin depletion, for example, you can take phenylalanine. As the precursor of noradrenalin and adrenalin, it is a natural remedy for depression. Tryptophan, as we've already seen, will replace the lost serotonin; glutamine, as well as regulating the blood sugar levels works as a brain fuel. Complementing the effects of the antidepressant phenylalanine, it banishes fatigue and promotes positive mental alertness.

Working together, these aminos help to relieve the mood disorders that are one of the most difficult aspects of alcoholism to treat. But amino acids can also be used to restore fluidity to cell walls. A blend of catabolic aminos (glycine, methionine and taurine) taken between 4 pm and 10 pm breaks down the cholesterol build-up that has taken place in the cell membranes to make them harder. This will help the neurotransmitters to connect effectively and enhance the effects of those mood-improving aminos, while a supplement of carnitine will help carry the excess fats to the mitochondria to be burnt.

Methionine and taurine are also used to help nurse the liver back to health when the scarring and fat build-up of cirrhosis has taken place.

Before we look at the formula which Geoff found so helpful let's briefly sum up what we've seen. As with every health problem alcoholism causes a variety of metabolic disorders, each of which tends to exaggerate the effects of the others. We've seen for instance what happens when alcohol in the blood lowers the blood sugar. As well as strengthening the craving for alcohol through the body's attempts to raise its blood sugar levels, drink also helps raise the circulating levels of leucine. This amino may in turn cause the kidneys to spill B3 and consequently deplete the body of tryptophan, serotonin and zinc (and in time their dependant co-factors) – causing mood-associated disorders, loss of enzymes and neurotransmitters, damaged capillaries and so on.

The effects of alcoholism range throughout the body and treating it means replacing each and every one of the nutrients that this awful, debilitating disease has stripped. Only then can an alcoholic reasonably expect to recover. And this is no idle theory. As Geoff and many others have proved amino acids and their co-factors do work. Here's the formulation he took:

Aminos
complete blend
glutamine
glycine
tryptophan
phenylalanine

Co-factors
B3
B12
C
zinc
selenium
catabolic aminos:
aspartic acid
methionine
taurine
(Best taken between 4 pm and 10 pm)

Chapter 20

Anorexia Aid

Anorexia nervosa is a frightening illness. The often extreme physical degeneration of the anorexic and his or her cunning and perverse ways of resisting help are daunting obstacles to overcome. In this illness, as for so many others, amino acid supplements can be an invaluable aid; more and more people affected by anorexia are turning to them for help.

Although some men and many adult women suffer from anorexia, girls in their early to mid-teens run the greatest risk of becoming anorexic. In Western Europe and North America as many as one girl in two hundred is now thought to be suffering from its effects. Often a throwaway comment about the shape of her body is enough to make a girl diet so excessively that she loses control. Or, as she enters puberty, she may experience fear at the powerful changes taking place in her body and try to escape them by starving herself. Because anorexics are often very bright, a desire to lose weight can be compounded by parental pressure to excel at school. She will feel she is being forced into a life over which she has no control. In the face of pressure like this, many girls see the habit of starvation as the only possible way of asserting their individuality. And this habit soon becomes an obsession.

The results are tragic; what little proteins an anorexic does eat are used with their co-factor nutrients simply to keep the body alive. In this life-or-death situation many non-essential bodily functions are sacrificed. The production of hormones for puberty is halted. Menstruation stops. The body quickly reverts to its pre-pubescent shape, losing a third or more of body weight in the process. The growth into womanhood is effectively arrested. Furthermore, an anorexic's self-perception will bcome hideously distorted. She will tell herself that she is happier and more in control. So, with enormous cunning, she will do all she can to maintain her weight loss.

Free-form amino acids supplements provide a sound nutritional base for recovery from the degeneration caused by the anorexia. By restoring normal functions to the metabolic pathways of the brain, they can alter the anorexic's self-perception, helping her to see her body, often for the first time, as it really is. Most important of all, they can actually make her want to get better.

Aminocide

In previous chapters we've seen how deficiencies of a single nutrient can affect the whole metabolic family. It's rather like flinging a stone into a pool of water; as it sinks it leaves a circular wave that expands to cover the whole surface of the pool. Now, instead of one stone, fling in a hundred, all at the same time, and it will give you some idea of the effects of anorexia. For an anorexic simply denies her body vital amounts of every nutrient that it needs to live. Accordingly, every single function of her body suffers. Zinc, for example, is vital in the manufacture of over eighty gut enzymes. Eating too little of just this one mineral prevents the small amounts of food which are eaten from being properly digested. The less nutrition the body absorbs, the fewer materials it will make available to create more digestive enzymes. (When an anorexic goes on one of her periodic and helpless binges the bloated sensation she feels afterwards is partly due to the gut's inability to digest what she's eaten.)

What this all means is that the amino acids which the body must have – to enable it to create hormones and neurotransmitters, repair cells, support the body's immune system, lay down bone tissue – when eaten at all are often left to putrefy in the gut. This in turn produces toxic by-products which, as we've seen, lead to food allergies, vulnerability to infection, fatigue and a variety of mental and emotional disturbances. Ironically, the metabolic pathways of an anorexic function at such a low ebb that there is often no use for many of the amino acids which do manage, against all the odds, to be absorbed. Instead they might be broken down and released as energy in the form of calories – the thing that anorexics fear most.

When the body's natural balance is so badly disrupted it will be subjected to almost continuous stress – functioning at the second, resistance, stage of the general adaptation syndrome (GAS). To support this stage, though, the body must have a complete and ample nutritional base. Yet anorexia destroys that base. If the two important amino acids in the stress response, phenylalanine and tyrosine, are depleted the body will use up greater quantities of vitamin C, itself needed to repair tissue and help all the amino acids which are absorbed to be used properly. Sooner or later an anorexic will succumb to the third stage of GAS – exhaustion. She will become even more susceptible to disease (anorexics are notoriously prone to glandular fever) and wounds will take much longer to heal. She will start to age prematurely - losing skin tone and hair condition. Her ability to concentrate will disappear. She will become easily agitated and frightened. All this in a body that, simply to survive, is forced to ravage itself, plundering its own muscles and fat supplies for the amino acids, vitamins and minerals it needs.

Precision Recovery

There is one widespread misconception among therapists treating anorexia - and in the ranks of general practitioners - and it highlights the advantages of using free-form amino acids. Put simply, they believe that re-educating an anorexic to eat, regardless of what is in her diet, is the most important objective.

It is not. It ignores the anorexic's inability to digest and utilize so much of what she eats. Often when she first starts eating again her stomach and small intestine lack the enzymes needed to break down the food. When this happens the body simply doesn't get the nutrients that are vital to strengthen the metabolic pathways. One result will be a painfully slow physical recovery. Another, and for an anorexic far worse, consequence will be a much too rapid weight increase. This is because of the damage anorexia causes to her endocrine organs. Many of the hormones these organs secrete, such as thyroxin and growth hormone, are necessary for the body to metabolize its food. Without these hormones a lot of her food will be converted immediately into calories and it will start to accumulate as fat. A runaway weight gain like this is the sort of trauma that causes a patient to relapse. So we can see that, despite the assertions of many anorexia therapists, specific details of an anorexic's diet are far from unimportant. In rehabilitating an anorexic they are absolutely essential.

Amino Supplementation

Amino acids help by assisting digestion and the functions of the metabolic pathways so that the patient's physical degeneration is arrested. In a recent study the amino acid levels of a hundred anorexics were examined. In each case their urinary amino acid profiles showed that they were low in every member of the amino acid family, together with most of the necessary co-factors. Each patient was put on a nutritional first-aid programme based on the complete free-form amino blend. In addition to the amino acids, vitamins C, B6 and E, calcium, iodine, magnesium and zinc were also prescribed to encourage efficient metabolization.

Because these amino acids are in their free-form states anorexics are able to absorb them. They pass straight through the gut and circulate to wherever they are needed. Arginine and ornithine, for example, generate production of growth hormone. This helps the body to employ its nutrients properly, metabolizing them into muscle and tissue structure. It also works to strengthen the immune system. Phenylalanine, on the other hand, enables the anorexic's body to respond to the stress demands. As the precursor of CCK, it acts on the hypothalamus as an appetite suppressant, lessening the anorexic's impulse to binge. Methionine and lysine combine to produce carnitine, which prevents sudden weight gain by mobilizing the fats in the blood to create energy. And, crucially, cysteine (the most prominent amino acid of the sex hormones FSH and LH) works with calcium to stimulate production of the major female sex hormone, estradiol, enabling the growth through puberty to resume. Amino acids also clear toxins from the system, reduce the stress placed on the body by the ravages of anorexia, help make the all-important digestive enzymes and are generally instrumental in promoting a return to full and balanced health.

The complete amino blend is attractive to anorexics because of its low calorie value. Taking such an all-inclusive supplement also spares them the stress of having to spend too much time deciding what to eat. Because of their high nutritional value they can be taken initially with smaller amounts of food than would otherwise be healthy, easing the anorexic more gently into the habit of eating solid food.

The Gargoyle Narcissus

Giving the anorexic physical support is important, but there is much more to the treatment than this. The disastrous effects on her body are only symptoms of the true nature of anorexia: a woeful misinterpretation by the anorexic of the internal and external stimuli of her life. When an anorexic looks in a mirror, standing face to face with the emaciated shadow of what she once was, all she sees is obesity. Stepping on to a weighing scale and finding she has gained a few ounces, all she feels is self-hatred. When she sees the increasing alarm of her friends and relations she cunningly diverts attention away from herself, often playing one person off against another, putting herself across as the wronged and defenceless party if people close to her try to be firm. Every aspect of her life becomes deadened by her morbid self-obsession.

Clearly anorexia stems from severe disturbances of the body image – disturbances which are created in the mind. Here too amino acids can prove immensely helpful, for amino acid supplements strengthen the metabolic pathways of the brain, helping alter mood, mental functioning and behaviour.

The Perception Aminos

A major cause of the mental and emotional disturbances of anorexia is thought to lie with imbalances in the brain's neurotransmitters. This is caused by an insufficient supply of specific amino acids. As we saw in earlier chapters neuro-transmitters are the chemicals which carry electrical brain messages between the nerve cells. Some neurotransmitters, like noradrenalin, are natural stimulants; others, like serotonin, have an inhibitory effect. Studies show that when serotonin levels are low people behave abnormally, often over-reacting to stimuli. Because of this, serotonin has been found effective in combating a variety of compulsive disorders, particularly the obsessive behaviour of anorexia.

The precursor of serotonin is the amino acid, tryptophan. As it is so much larger than other amino molecules it often has difficulty competing for absorption with other, smaller, amino acids. Most people's tryptophan levels are generally quite low. Because protein foods often divert tryptophan to other metabolic tasks, eating a protein-free meal actually makes tryptophan more available to the brain. Anorexics need all the protein they can get, though, so additional doses of tryptophan are often prescribed on top of the amounts contained in the full blend.

Another substance found to be effective in helping the brain functions of anorexics is glutamine. Once across the protective blood brain barrier it is converted into its less mobile amino form, glutamic acid. It is not a neurotransmitter but, with the blood sugar glucose, aids brain function as a brain fuel. It has been used by physicians and nutritionists in lessening cravings, fighting mental disorders and eliminating the toxic waste-product ammonia. It is also an excellent remedy for fatigue.

Finally, we come to the amino acid, asparagine. Along with glutamic acid it is the most commonly found amino in the brain. As it is present in such high quantities researchers think it must play a major role in maintaining optimum brain function, helping to regulate the metabolism of the brain and cells of the nervous system. In fact, people with emotional and behavioural problems almost invariably suffer from low levels of asparagine. In a recent test 150 out of 152 patients experiencing severe emotional and behavioural disorders were found to have levels of asparagine well below the norm. When it was given to them as a supplement all the patients reported a growth in self-confidence and an increased desire to face the problems of their lives head-on.

A good dosage of these three aminos is 500 mg of each, three times a day, together with 40 mg each of vitamins B1 and B2 and 200 mg of folic acid. To prevent competition with other amino acids, allowing them to reach the brain, these doses should ideally be spaced equally between meals and the full blend. Better still, taking them with some carbohydrate – like a slice of wholemeal bread – greatly encourages brain take-up.

Happy Endings

More and more people whose lives have been ruined by anorexia are now turning to amino acids for help. Mary was a 29-year-old nurse who had waged an on and off battle with anorexia since her mid-teens. Over a period of about twelve years she had visited six psychiatrists. After each course of treatment she staged a recovery, only to relapse back into her anorexic obsessions after two months or so. She had never menstruated fully. Despite her starved appearance, looking years beyond her age, she denied that she felt particularly ill. She was immediately put on the full amino blend, together with additional tryptophan and glutamine – only agreeing to take them because of their low calorie values.

After only a few days of taking the supplements the change in her attitude was astonishing: 'I looked in the mirror and was stunned to see how horribly thin I was. My perceptions had changed overnight. All that time when I was convinced of my obesity I was actually little more than a scarecrow.' With a new-found sense of lucidity giving her the determination to recover, she started a wholefood diet supplemented by free-form amino acids and their co-factors. Within three months she was healthier than she'd been in her life.

Lois was a 41-year-old woman who had been made to seek help by her worried son. She denied that there was anything seriously wrong with her and she was noncommital and secretive when questioned about her anorexia. After taking the complete blend for less than a week she confessed that she was bulemic (making herself sick after she ate) as well as anorexic and had been so for almost twenty years! In the last five years the illness had progressively worsened. She had lost her job and her husband had left her. She felt constantly on the verge of a nervous breakdown and suffered from insomnia, lack of concentration and extreme fatigue.

As well as the full amino blend, she was given extra asparagine, tryptophan and glutamine, together with their co-factors. Within a very short while she had staged a remarkable recovery. She felt strong and full of physical energy. Furthermore she was mentally composed and alert – a stark contrast with her former unfocused and hyperactive state of mind, so characteristic of anorexia. She met her second husband soon after on a skiing holiday in Italy.

As encouraging as these examples are, the disturbing fact is that these women, both well into adulthood, had been anorexic since their teens. They had repeatedly sought help and been treated by psychiatrists whose attitude seemed to be: 'Get them used to eating and the battle is won.' In many, less severe, cases this approach probably works, but it's a desperately hit-or-miss affair. Most anorexics who do recover admit to 'constantly having to look over my shoulder, knowing that the spectre of anorexia is still there'. Not surprisingly, many suffer a relapse. Getting the anorexic to start eating and then simply hoping for the best is not the answer, as Mary and Lois will testify. Sadly, there seems to be a gulf between the therapists' aims, which are to help the anorexic to recover, and their methods, which are to feed her with literally anything that comes to hand.

Free-form amino acids can bridge that gulf. They supply in a concentrated and balanced form all the nutrients an anorexic needs to recover physiologically. At the same time they help the brain to work properly. Striking at the very heart of the illness, they can restore a patient's balance, perception and lucidity.

Final Words

In this book we've not only tried to illustrate the nutritional value of free form amino acids but also explained how you can use them to their best advantage. This has often meant exploring the workings of the body's metabolic pathways. Perhaps at times this maze of interlocking biochemical routes – where following the changes wrought on one amino as it reacts with enzymes and co-factors inevitably leads you to the way that others are changed in turn – has seemed confusing to you. If so just remember that any maze can confuse only as long as you don't know your way around it. Once you have a map you can get about with ease, what seemed baffling appears childishly simple and the new-found familiarity allows you to reach your destination. In the same way, understanding your way round the metabolic pathways – knowing which 'turning' you must take to reach a particular goal – enables you to start actively raising your level of wellbeing. Of course, choosing a turning in this case means knowing which amino supplements to use so that a metabolic pathway can function at peak performance. That's where this book comes in.

We've explained the importance to your health of individual reactions in the body, showing which aminos are responsible and listing blends of aminos and co-factors which are most effective at allowing the reactions to occur. The riches this approach offers in terms of your health makes 'The Amino Revolution' something of a treasure map. You've seen what it has meant for the victims of a wide variety of health disorders – from mental and emotional problems such as stress, depression and anorexia to physical difficulties which have included infertility, allergies and viruses. All that remains is for you to follow the 'map' yourself the next time you should need it. When you do, simply remember that with their ability to penetrate right to the heart of the difficulty free-form amino acids are unsurpassed in their health-enhancing potential.

The remaining pages offer some additional advice on how to get the best from your amino supplements.

Appendix I

At-a-Glance Guide to Amino Supplementation

This list outlines the aminos you can take to help relieve a specific health problem – mental, emotional or physical. Referring to it when you are unwell will help you to decide on a blend which is best for you.

First, let's look at the conditions which are helped by taking the complete amino blend:

Anorexia
Slimming on a low protein diet
Stress
Pre- and post-operative support
Strengthening immune system – against frequent colds, infections etc.
Cancer – when there is a need for extremely high amounts of protein
Vegetarian diet – as a safeguard measure
Body-building
Digestive problems
Brittle nails
Hair loss
Dizziness
Cold intolerance
Hypotension (low blood pressure)

Men should take a maximum of 15 grammes of the complete blend three times a day and women should take a maximum of 10 grammes three times a day. The minimum dosage is usually two grammes a day.

Now let's look at the conditions which warrant attention with individual amino acid supplementation:

Alcoholism:
glutamine
tryptophan
cysteine
methionine (for cirrhosis of the liver)

Allergies:
cysteine
histidine

Angina:
carnitine
taurine

Anxiety:
tyrosine
histidine
glycine
taurine
tryptophan

Appetite control:
phenylalanine

Arthritis:
histidine
cysteine
glycine
glutathione

Brittle nails:
cysteine

Chronic pain:
DL-phenylalanine
tryptophan
glycine

Depression:
glutamine
phenylalanine
tyrosine
tryptophan

Difficulty in achieving orgasm:
histidine

Drug addiction:
phenylalanine
tyrosine
tryptophan
glutamine

Exposure to heavy metals:
glutathione
methionine

Exposure to radiation:
tyrosine
methionine
histidine
glutathione

Fatigue:
glutamine
phenylalanine
methionine
lysine
arginine

Hair loss:
cysteine

Herpes:
lysine
methionine

Hypertension:
histidine
tryptophan
taurine

Hypoglycemia:
glycine
lysine
glutamine

Inability to concentrate:
glutamine
lysine
phenylalanine

Infertility:
arginine
carnitine

Insomnia:
tryptophan

Loss of libido:
phenylalanine

Loss of memory:
methionine
arginine
ornithine

Low blood pressure:
tyrosine
phenylalanine

Low stomach acid:
glutamic acid HCL
betaine HCL
histidine

Peptic ulcer:
glutamine
histidine

Premature ejaculation:
methionine

Poor circulation:
carnitine
taurine

Skin problems:
cysteine
glutathione

Slow healing:
arginine
ornithine
cysteine
leucine

Smoking:
tryptophan
histidine
glutamine
phenylalanine

Tremors:
glycine
taurine
phenylalanine
tyrosine
tryptophan

Individual amino acids are best taken in doses of between 250 mg and 1500 mg a day. It's best not to exceed the higher dosage without guidance from a doctor or health practitioner.

Appendix II

Safety and Precautions

In their bestselling health book *Life Extension*, Durk Pearson and Sandy Shaw devote an entire chapter to the possible dangers of nutritional supplementation. The chapter, entitled 'Is there anything perfectly safe?' consists of one word: NO.

The fact is no matter what you give your body there is always an element of risk involved. Amino acids are the building blocks of protein. As food proteins are part of our daily diet, free-form amino acid supplements are relatively safe. But in some patients even these may cause the occasional side-effect. In this chapter we'll underline the precautions you should always take when using the free-form powders and itemize the adverse reactions which have sometimes been known to occur.

Put a Blend to It All

As we've seen, each of the fifty thousand or more proteins in your body has its own unique amino acid profile. The number, selection and sequence of amino acids they contain differs from one protein to the next. This is what gives them their versatility and allows the body to reconstruct them wherever, and in whatever form, it needs them. In a normal, healthy body this presents no problem. Your body synthesizes the proteins in the pancreas, liver or muscles, or dips directly into the pool of circulating aminos. As its needs vary from day to day, aminos which the body doesn't want are simply broken down and used as energy. Every one of your body's functions – from manufacturing muscle and creating enzymes to tearing apart unwanted protein – takes place in stage-by-stage reactions called metabolic pathways. The first, and most important precaution when you take free-form amino acids is simply to remember this fact.

Your food enters the metabolic pathways almost from the moment you swallow it. Enzymes break the protein down into its individual amino acids which your body then uses to meet its astonishingly long list of needs – transforming them into skin tissue, enzymes, hormones, neurotransmitters, hair and bone structure. Illnesses occur when something blocks a transformation causing the metabolic pathway to work sluggishly. Taking a free-form amino acid helps to relieve your illness by unblocking the pathway and allowing the transformations to take place.

Now we're coming to the crunch. Let's imagine you're using a particular free-form amino to unblock a pathway which caused an illness. What you might have forgotten to consider is that the pathway which you've decided to supplement meets and reacts with many others. No metabolic pathway in your body proceeds in isolation. Therefore, using an amino acid to alter this one naturally alters those others which cross it. This might be a good thing. It often sets off a synergistic wave that helps to strengthen many connected pathways as well as the one you were concentrating on. But suppose for a minute that a second pathway was adversely affected by the way you supplemented the first. Perhaps the productivity of the first increases so that the second suddenly finds itself having to convert more of a particular substance. What if this second pathway was itself a little sluggish, perhaps due to an enzyme depletion? Not enough to cause a recognizable illness but, unable to convert all it receives, enough to cause a build-up of the chemical which the rejuvenated first pathway has sent it. What you get then is a metabolic traffic jam.

This means that the body, in trying to cope with the increased load on this pathway, will divert vitamins and minerals needed for other functions to help deal with the unconverted substances. This will put strains on other parts of the body and, in time, cause other pathways to break down. Your immune system might perform less efficiently; you might not be able to respond to stress so well; you might get tired and feel weak. You might even become more ill than you were before you took the supplement.

The key to ensuring this doesn't happen is not to take a supplement of a single amino acid, but rather one of the blends included in this book. Together, of course, with the vitamins and minerals the body uses to convert them fully in the metabolic pathways. Taking these nutrients in groups insures your body against the sort of overload and stresses that a single amino might cause.

This isn't an unbreakable rule that we're applying. We're not saying that a single amino will cause the problems we've just mentioned, nor that amino acids are any more dangerous than other supplements such as vitamins (most of them are even safer than the benign vitamin C). Indeed many people benefit immensely from using a single amino acid to help them recover from a disorder. Nonetheless, we do recommend that you take formulas whose constituent aminos, vitamins and minerals complement each other such as those included in the blends we've mentioned. After all, the truth behind orthomolecular nutrition is that the best route towards full health and vitality lies in giving the body an optimal and balanced supply of all it needs – rather than just 'pumping up' the area that requires the most obvious attention. This is also another excellent reason for taking doses of the complete blend in addition to those more specifically designed formulations. This awareness of your body as an interdependent whole is the most important safety measure that you can possess. There are a few warnings to give about using amino acids in particular circumstances and we'll look at these next.

Phenylketonuria

The first precaution is that you should never take DL or L-phenylalanine if you are a phenylketonuric. Phenylketonuria is a genetic inability to manufacture the enzyme which converts phenylalanine to tyrosine. It is particularly dangerous during the first four years of life when, unless the intake of naturally occuring phenylalanine is controlled, it will build up and cause mental retardation. No matter how old you are, though, if you suffer from this problem you shouldn't take phenylalanine.

Genetic problems like this are very rare. But they do exist and new ones may be discovered. If you have difficulty metabolizing a particular amino acid you may suffer by taking free-form supplements. You might not realize you have a problem until unpleasant physical or psychological symptoms occur. If this happens stop taking your amino supplements immediately and only start again under the direction of a health practitioner.

MAO inhibitors

Certain amino acids should be avoided when taking mono-amino oxidase (MAO) inhibitors, the man-made antidepressants prescribed under many different names. They work by inhibiting the enzyme MAO which is responsible for deactivating the catecholamines (noradrenalin and adrenalin) and serotonin after use. This inhibiting effect causes these substances to circulate in the body for much longer than usual, helping to relieve depression, anxiety and stress. The bad side is that MAO inhibitors also cause severe depletion of many essential nutrients and have been known to lead to anorexia among other problems.

If you take phenylalanine, tyrosine or tryptophan with MAO inhibitors the surge in the levels of circulating adrenalin, noradrenalin and serotonin the combination would cause could lead to a range of mood-related and psychotic problems. Because of this you should only take one or the other – never both. We've seen many times in the book how and why these three aminos are so much better for your health than MAO inhibitors. If you are taking MAO inhibitors now, instead of having to avoid free-form amino acids, why not do without the inhibitors?

Digestion

Since free-form amino acids have no fibre or bulk and are absorbed immediately they may have a mild constipating effect. However, if you eat well, particularly lots of fresh fruit and vegetables, it's a problem you're not likely to encounter. If, on the other hand, you take a mega-dose of an amino acid (a very rare fifteen grammes or more) it might cause diarrhoea.

L-Arginine

As we saw in chapter 11 laboratory tests suggest that the growth of herpes can be stimulated by arginine .Some nutritionists feel that in practice it may not do this as it has many other effects in the body, one of which is to strengthen the immune system. However, if you have herpes it's worth avoiding arginine and substituting ornithine in its place.

L-Aspartic acid

May cause flatulence!

Branched-chain aminos

Always take these three – leucine, isoleucine and valine – together in a blend unless you wish deliberately to cut down or increase the body's intake of one of them. Excess leucine, for example, causes the kidneys to spill vitamin B3. You can counter this by taking extra amounts of isoleucine or B3.

Carnitine

You may see the DL version of this amino on sale in health food shops. If so, make sure that it's the version you want. You will remember that L-carnitine mobilizes fat deposits and is an important part of amino therapy for slimming and heart disease. The 'DL' version, however, antagonizes L-carnitine, preventing fat metabolism from taking place.

L-Cysteine

The general reccomendation when using cysteine (to relieve skin complaints, for example) is to take three times the amount of vitamin C with it. Vitamin C prevents the cysteine oxidizing to cystine, an amino which won't help you in the same way.

Gamma-Aminobutyric-Acid (GABA)

In tests Carl Pfeiffer discovered that in some individuals ten grammes of this calming amino can be mildly discomforting. It may cause nausea, your skin to flush and perhaps a headache.

L-Histidine

Doses of four grammes and above of histidine taken in one go have been known to cause early menstruation. Because of this some women athletes use it to time their periods away from important sporting events. A few people have unnaturally high histamine levels, and in a fraction it causes schizophrenic tendencies. This excess histamine is probably created by putrefaction in the gut because of poor digestion rather than the histidine from their food. Nevertheless people with a history of schizophrenia should seek advice before taking free form supplements of histidine.

L-Methionine

Some nutritionists have reported that an excess of this amino may result in psychological problems. This is more probably due to a shortage of magnesium, which is low in most people and is the substance methionine needs in the first stage of its metabolic pathways. Whenever you take methionine simply make sure that you have adequate magnesium. It's also a good idea to drink at least a pint of water a day when you are taking methionine.

DL-Phenylalanine

As this relieves chronic pain so effectively it's the only 'DL' form of an amino acid that we recommend you take. If you suffer from high hypertension, only take DLPA under a doctor's or nutritionist's direction and have your blood pressure monitored regularly. If you take MAO inhibitors follow the advice we gave you about them on page 192.

L-Phenylalanine and L-Tyrosine

Likewise, avoid these two if you suffer from high blood pressure.

None of these warnings may apply to you, and even if one does it's the easiest thing in the world to stop taking the offending amino acid supplement. The only safety precaution that we do stress is that you balance the aminos with their co-factors. In a way this is less of a precaution and more of an attitude. Because when you realize that illness doesn't stem from an isolated cause any more than you can treat that illness with a solitary medicine or supplement you are taking the first step into a healthier and more vital life.

Appendix III

Sources of Amino Acid Products

When you decide to buy free form amino acids make sure that it's from a company that is willing to disclose their formulations to you. If they are not listed on the cannister label then the supplier should be able to give you a list of the ingredients upon request. Often blends or mixtures are loaded with some of the more inexpensive amino acids and even protein (peptide) powders then sold at a tremendous mark-up.

Amino acids are becoming more widely available from health food stores under a variety of different brand names. Many are sold in convenient blends of two or more separate aminos. Read the container thoroughly before buying to make sure that all you get is unadulterated free-form aminos. If you can't find a shop near you that sells them here are some addresses of good suppliers and stockists:

Cantassium
Larkhall Laboratories
225 Putney Bridge Road
London SW15
(01) 870 0971

Natural Flow
Burwash Common
East Sussex
(0435) 882482

Nature's Best
P.O. Box 1
Tunbridge Wells
Kent TN2 3EQ
(0892) 34143
(For health practitioners only, write to Lamberts at the same address)

Nature's Own
Cheltenham GI50 1HX

Appendix IV

Urinary Amino Tests

Since urinary amino tests are quite expensive, we are breaking our list of sources of such tests into two parts. The first part gives the addresses of clinics or laboratories that use sulpho-salycilic acid as part of their measurement test; the second gives the addresses which use HCL. Since HCL acts differently, by breaking down glutamine into glutamic acid and glutamic acid into its constituents, we recommend sulpho-salycilic acid sources as our first choice.

Sources of urinary amino acid tests using sulpho-salycilic acid as the deproteinizer and preservative of the urine sample:

Great Britain
Medabolics Limited
14 Mount Pleasant Road
Tunbridge Wells
Kent TN1 1QU
(0892) 42609

York Medical Laboratories
York

Netherlands
European Laboratory of Nutrients
Gebouw MPPC
J M Kemperstraat 3
3581 K G Utrecht
(3405) 64260

Australia
Xandria Williams
366 Military Road
Cremorne 2090
290 4771

USA
Medabolics
22318 N.E. 169th Street
Brush Prairie
WA 98606
(206) 254 2202
(outside Washington (800) 257 1121)

Sources of tests using HCL:

USA
Smith Klyne
Bio-Science Laboratories
7600 Tyrone Avenue
Van Nuys
CA 91405

Doctor's Data
30 W. 101
Roosevelt Road
West Chicago
ILL 60195

Appendix V

References

Chapter 1
Ajinomoto Co., *Amino Acids* (Part 3), Tokyo, 1980
Chaitow L., *Amino Acids in Therapy*, Thorsons, New York, 1985
Greerstein J. and Winitz M., *Chemistry of Amino Acids*, Wiley, New York, 1931
Guyton A., *Textbook of Medical Physiology*, 5th edition, Saunder, 1976
Meister A., *Biochemistry of Amino Acids*, 2nd edition, Academic Press, New York, 1965
Rose S., *The Chemistry of Life*, Pelican, London, 1985

Chapter 2
Bremer H. and others, *Disturbances of Amino Acid Metabolism: Clinical Chemistry and Diagnosis*, Urban and Schwarzenberg, Baltimore, 1981
Lehninger A., *Biochemistry: the Molecular Basis of Cell Structure and Function*, Worth Publishers, New York, 1970
McGilvery R., *Biochemistry: a Functional Approach*, Saunders, London, 1970
Meiss D., and others, 'Amino Acid Analysis: an Important Nutritional and Clinical Evaluation Tool', *Nutr. Perspectives*, 6 (2) 1983, 19-24
Rattenbury, J., *Amino Acid Analysis*, Halsted Press, 1981
Salaman M., 'Amino Acid Testing', *Let's Live*, Aug. 1984, 82-3
Stryer, L., *Biochemistry*, Freeman Co, San Francisco, 1975

Chapter 3
Bender D., *Amino Acid Metabolism*, Wiley, 1985
Colgen M., *Your Personal Vitamin Profile*, Quill, New York, 1982
Devlin T., *Textbook of Biochemistry with Clinical Applications*, Wiley, 1982
Jo-Mar Laboratories 'Introduction to the Amazing Amino Acids with their strange-sounding names', Los Gatos, California, 1981, Booklet 1
Munro H. and Crim M., 'The proteins and amino acids' in *Modern Nutrition in Health and Disease*, edited by Goodhart and Shils, 5th edition, 1978

Chapter 4
Ader R. (ed.), *Psychoneuroimmunology*, Academic Press, New York, 1981
Barchas J. and others, 'Behavioral Neurochemistry: Neuroregulators and Behavioral States, *Science 200*, May 26, 1976, 964-73

Bender D., *Amino Acid Metabolism*, Wiley, 1985

Bland J., *Medical Applications of Clinical Nutrition*, Keats, 1983

Butter C., *Neuropsychology; the Study of Brain and Behavior*, Brooks/Cole, 1969

Cooper J. and others, *The Biochemical Basis of Neuropharmacology*, Oxford Press, 1978

Curson G. (ed.), *The Biochemistry of Psychiatric Disturbances*, Wiley, 1980

DeFeudis, 'Amino Acids as Central Neurotransmitters, *Ann. Res. Pharmacol*, 15, 1975, pp105-127

Fernstrom J., 'Effects of Precursors on Brain Neurotransmitter Synthesis and Brain Functions', *Dia betologia*, 1981, 20:281-89

Frank B., *Dr Frank's No-Ageing Diet*, Dial Press, 1978

Green A. and Costain D., *Pharmacology and Biochemistry of Psychiatric Disorders*, Wiley, 1981

Hawkins D. and Pauling L., *Orthomolecular Psychiatry*, Freeman, San Francisco, 1973

Hoffa A. 'Mega Amino Acid Therapy', *Ortho. Psych.* Vol. 9, 1983, pp2-5

Iverson L. and others, *Handbook of Psychopharmacology*, Plenum Press, 1978

Longo V. F., *Neuropharmacology and Behavior*, Freeman, 1972

Passwater R., 'Notes on Stress, Heart Attacks and Problems of the Mind', *Health Quarterly Journal*, Vol. 5 Nov-Dec, 1980

Pfeiffer C., *Mental and Elemental Nutrients*, Keats, 1975

Quastel J., 'The role of Amino Acids in the Brain', essays in *Medical Biochemistry*, Vol. 4, London, 1979

Reichelt and Kyamme, 'Acetylated and Peptide bound Glutamate and Aspartate in the Brain', *Journal of Neurochemistry*, 14, 1967, 987

Seiden L. and Dykstra L., *Psychopharmacology: a Biochemical and Behavioural Approach*, Van Nostrand, 1977

Watson G., *Nutrition and your Mind: the Psychochemical Response*, Harper and Row, London, 1972

Chapter 5

Barbul and others, 'Arginine, a Thymotropic and Wound-healing Promoting Agent', *Surgical Forum*, 28: 1977, 101-103

Beisel W.R., 'Malnutrition as a consequence of stress', in *Malnutrition and the Immune Responses*, Suskind (ed.), Raven Press, New York, 1977

Blackburn and others, 'Branched Chained Amino Acids Administration and Metabolism during Starvation, Injury and Infection.' *Surgery 86*, 1979, 307-15

Border and others, 'Multiple Systems Organ Failure: Muscle fuel deficit with visceral Protein Malnutrition,' *Surgery 56*, 1976, 1147-50

Cerra and others, 'Septic Autocannibalism: a Failure of Exogeneous Nutritional Support', *Ann. Surgery*, 1980

Cerra F. and others, 'Branched Chains Support Postoperative Protein Synthesis,' *Surgery 92*, 1982, 192-9

Cuthbertson D. and others, 'Metabolism during the Post Injury Period,' *Adv. Clin. Chem.* 1969, 12211-55

Waterlow J. and others, 'The Measurement of Rates of Protein Turnover, Synthesis and Breakdown in Man and the Effects of Nutritional Status and Surgical Injury,' *American Journal of Nutrition* 30, 1977, 1933-39

Chapter 6
Barchas J. and others, 'Behavioral Neurochemistry, Neuroregulators and Behavioral States', *Science* 200 May 26, 1978, 964-73

Cherkin A. & Van Harreveld A., 'L-Proline and Related Compounds: Correlation of Structure Amnesic Potency and Anti-spreading Depression Potency', *Brain Research* 156, 1978, 265-73

Geldenberg A. and others, 'Tyrosine for Treatment of Depression', *Am. J. of Psychiatry*, 137, 1980, 622-3

Goldberg I., 'L-Tyrosine in Depression', *Lancet* 2, 1980, 364

Hawkins D. & Pauling L., *Orthomolecular Psychiatry*, Freeman, San Francisco, 1973

Pearson D. & Shaw S. *Life Extension*, Warner, 1982

Pearson D. & Shaw S., *The Life Extension Companion*, Warner, 1984

Rose W. and others, 'The Amino Acid Requirements of Man. The Phenylalanine Requirement', *J. Biol. Chem.* 213, 1955, 913-22

Chapter 7
Cheraskin & Ringsdorf, 'Psychodietetics' Bantam, New York, 1976

Ellis J. and others, 'Flight Induced Changes in Human Amino Acid Excretion', *Aviation, Space and Environment Med.* 1-8, Jan, 1976

Growdon J.H. & Wurtman R, 'Dietary influences on the synthesis of neurotransmitters in the brain', *Nutr. Rev.* 37, 1979, 129-36

Hale H. and others, 'Human Amino Acid Excretion Patterns During and Following Prolonged Multistressor tests', *Aviation, Space and Environmental Med.*, Feb. 1975, 173-8

Hawkins P. and others, 'Amino Acid supply to Individual Cerebral Structures in Awake and Anesthetized Rats', *Amer. Physiol. Soc.* E1-11, 1982

Hoffer, 'Orthomolecular Nutrition', Keats, Connecticut, 1978

Chapter 8
Bland J., *Medical Applications of Clinical Nutrition*, Keats, 1983

Lessor M., *Nutrition and Vitamin Therapy*, Grove Press, New York, 1980

Scriver C. & Rosenberg L., *Amino Acid Metabolism and its disorders*, W.B. Saunders, 1973

Stanbury J. and others, *The Metabolic Basis of Inherited Disease*, McGraw Hill, 1978

Williams R., *Nutrition against disease*, Bantam Books, 1981

Chapter 9
Lessor M., *Nutrition and Vitamin Therapy*, Grove Press, New York, 1980

Mann T., *The biochemistry of Semen and the Male Reproductive Tract*, Wiley, 1964

Pfeiffer C., *Mental and Elemental Nutrients*, Keats, 1975

Pryor J. and others, 'Controlled Clinical trial of Arginine for Infertile Men with Oligozoospermin, *Br. T. Urol*, 50(1), Feb 1978, 47-50

Chapter 10
Shive W. and others, 'Glutamine in the treatment of peptic ulcer', *Texas State J. of Medicine*, Vol. 53, 1957, 640-3
'The importance of gastrointestinal pH balance', *Bulletin of Heidelberg International*, Norcross, Georgia, USA, 30092

Chapter 11
Griffith R. and others, 'A Multicentred Study of Lysine Therapy in Herpes Simplex Infection', *Dermatologica* 156(5), 1978, 256-67
Milman N. and others, 'Lysine Prophylaxis in recurrent Herpes Simplex Labialic', *Acta Dorm Venereol*, (Stockh) 60, 1980, 85-7
Sanchez A. and others, 'Plasma Amino Acids in Human Fed Plant Proteins', *Nutritional Reports International*, Sept 1983, 497-507

Chapter 12
Levine S. & Kidd P., *Antioxidant Adaptation*, Allergy Research Group, San Leandro Ca, 1985
Phillpot W. & Kalita D., *Brain Allergies*, Keats, 1981
Phillpot W. & Kalita D., *Victory over Diabetics*, Keats, 1983

Chapter 13
Barbul and others, 'Thymotropic Actions of Arginine, Ornithine and Growth Hormone', *Fed. Proc.*, 1978, 282
Butler R. and others, 'The effects of preloads of amino acids on short-term satiety', *American Journal of Clinical Nutrition*, Oct 1982, 2045-7
Fox A., *The Beverly Hills Medical Diet*, Bantam Books, 1981
Isidori and others, 'A Study of Growth Hormone Release in Man after Oral Administration of Amino Acids', *Curr. Med. Res. Opi.*, 475-81
Kenton L., *Biogenic Diet*, Century, 1986
Koppf and others, 'Plasma Growth Hormone Response to Intravenous Administration of Amino Acids', *J. Clin. Endocr.* 25, 1985, 1140-4
McDougall J. and M., *The McDougall Plan*, New Century Publishers
Merinee and others, 'Arginine initiated Release of Human Growth Hormone', *New Engl. J. Med.*, 183(26), 1969, 1425-9
Newbold H., *Dr. Newbold's Revolutionary New Discoveries About Weight Loss*, Rawson Assoc. 1977
Passwater R., *Supernutrition For a Healthy Heart*, Dial Press, 1977
Pearson and Shaw, *The Life Extension Weight Loss Programme*, Doubleday, 1986
Scriver C. and Rosenbury L., *Amino Acid Metabolism and its Disorders*, Saunders, Philadelphia, 1973
Wade C., *The New Enzyme Catalyst Diet*, Parker Publishing, 1976
Williams R., *Nutrition Against Disease*, Bantam Books, 1981

Chapter 14

Bland J., *Medical Applications of Clinical Nutrition*, Keats, 1983
Journal of American Medical Association Dec 15, 1978, 2712-4
Pearson and Shaw, *Life Extension*, Warner, 1982
'Proteins', *Nutrition Reports International*, Sept 1983, 497-507
Sanchez A. and others, 'Plasma Amino Acids in Humans',
Sved A. and others, 'Studies on the Antihypertensive Action of L-tryptophan', *J. of Pharm and Exp.* Therapeutic Vol. 221, 1982, 329-33

Chapter 15

Blackburn and others, *Amino Acids*, John Wright, 1983
Davidson A. and others, 'Brain Decarboxylase Activities as Indices of Pathological Change in Senile Dementia', *Lancet*, 1974, 1247
Hoffer A. and Walker M., *Nutrients to Age Without Senility*, Keats, 1980
Kenton L., *Ageless Ageing*, Century, 1985
Levine S. and Kidd P., *Antioxidant Adaptation*, Allergy Research Group, San Leandro, California, 1985
Lundholm K., 'Ageing Amino Acid and Protein Metabolism'
Wade C., *Miracle Protein*, Parker Publishing, New York, 1975

Chapter 16

Bondy P. and Rosenberg l., *Metabolic Control and Disease*, Saunders 8th ed., Philadelphia, 1980
Stryer L., *Biochemistry*, S.H. Freeman, San Francisco, 1975

Chapter 17

Sprince H. and others, 'Comparison of Protection by L-Ascorbic Acid, L-Cysteine, and Adrenergic-Blocking Agents Against Acetaldehyde, Acrolein, and Formaldehyde Toxicity, Implications in Smoking.' *Agents and Actions* 9, 1979, 407

Chapter 18

Ikeda H., 'Effects of Taurine on Alcohol Withdrawal' *Lancet* Sept. 1977, 509
Lowry M., *Under The Volcano*, Penguin, London, 1983
Morgan M. and others, 'Ratio of Plasma Amino-n-Butyric Acid to Leucine as an Empirical Marker of Alcoholism', *Science*, Sept 16, 1977, 1183-5
Ravel J. and others, 'Reversal of Alcohol Toxicity by Glutamine', *Journ. Biol. Chem.*, Vol. 214, 1955, 497-501
Rogers L., 'Some Biological Effects of Glutamine', *Am. Chem. Soc.* Houston, Dec 1955
Rogers L. and Pelton, 'Glutamine in the Treatment of Alcoholism', *Quarterly Jour. of Studies on Alcohol*, Vol. 18, no. 4, 1957
Trunnel J. and Wheeler J., 'Preliminary Report on Experiments with Orally Administered Glutamine Treatment in Treatment of Alcoholics', *Am. Chem. Soc.*, Dec 1955
Williams R., *Alcoholism: The Nutritional Approach*, Univ. of Texas, 1959

Chapter 19

Newbold H., *Mega-Nutrients For Your Nerves*, Peter Wyden Press, New York 1975

Quastel J., 'The Role of Amino Acids in the Brain', essays in *Medical Biochemistry*, Vol. 4, Great Britain, 1979, 1-48

Reinis S. and Goldman J., *The Chemistry of Behavior*, Plenum Press, New York, 1982

Wurtman R., 'Nutrients That Modify Brain Function', *Scientific Amer.* April 1982

Chapter 20

Bender D., *Amino Acid Metabolism*, 2nd edition, Wiley, 1985

Blackburn and others (eds.), *Amino Acid Metabolism and Medical Applications*, John Wright, 1983

Cunningham-Rundles S., 'Effects of Nutritional Status on Immunological Function', *Amer. Jour. of Clin. Nutr.* May 1982, 1202-10

Wright J. and Gaby A., 'Clinical Applications of Nutritional Biochemistry', Seminar, San Francisco, 1983

Appendix II – Safety and Precautions

'Adaptive Responses of Amino Acid Degrading Enzymes to Variations of Amino Acid and Protein Intake', *Nutritional Reviews*, Nov 1976

Filer L.J. and others, 'Plasma Amino-Grams in Infants and Adults Fed an Identical High Protein Meal', *Fed Prog.* 36, 1977, 1181

Forbes A., 'Regulation of Oral Amino Acid Preparations', *Clinical Nutritional Update*, Amer. Medic. Assoc., Chicago, 1977

Harper A.E. and others, 'Effects of Ingestion of Disproportionate Amounts of Amino Acids', *Physiol. Rev.* 50, 1970, 428

Reynolds W.A. and others, 'Monosodium Glutamate: Absence of Hypothalamic Lesions After Ingestion by Newborn Primates', *Science* 172, 1971, 1342

Stegink L.D., 'Absorption, Utilization and Safety of Aspartic Acid', *J. Toxicol, and Environ, Health*, 2, 1976, 215

Snyderman S., 'Levels of the Anomalies of Amino Acid Metabolism', *Amino Acids Clinical Nutrition Update American Medical Association*, Chicago, 1977, 159-166

Index

acne, 148
actin, 7
adaptive energy, 46
adrenalin, 10, 15, 24, 47, 54
ageing, 135-43
ageing formula, 143
alcohol, 16, 27
alcoholism, 169-77, 186
alcoholism formula, 177
allergy, 30, 106-13, 186
allergy formula, 113
amino acids, 5
ammonia, 15, 38, 48, 59
anabolic cycle, 77
angina, 27, 129, 187
anorexia nervosa, 178-84, 186
anxiety, 29, 61-7, 187
anxiety formula, 66
appetite control, 187
arginine, 23, 28, 32, 43, 50, 76, 80, 82, 83, 121, 142, 154
arteriosclerosis, 41, 127
arthritis, 27, 141, 187
asparagine, 31, 182
aspartic acid, 142
Astbury, W., 7
axon, 36, 54

B-cell antibody, 76
Bacques, D., 167
BCAA, 28
betaine, 92
biofeedback, 100
blood brain barrier, 55
blood pressure, low, 24, 189
boils, 148
branched chain aminos, 28, 193
brain, 35-6

Brain Bio Centre, Princeton, 40
brittle nails, 187
bronchitis, 27

calcium, 28, 30
calcium phosphate, 7
cancer, 140-141
candida albicans, 73
cantassium, 195
carbohydrates, 5
carbon, 6
carboxypeptase, 74
carnitine, 28, 76, 118, 129, 130, 134, 168, 176, 193
catabolic cycle, 77
catecholamines, 23, 24, 54, 57
CCK, 116, 168
chelation therapy, 132-4
chelators, anti-ageing, 141
Cheraskin, Dr, 64, 89
cholesterol, 5
choline, 129
cholycystokinin, 116, 168
chymotrypsin, 74
cigarette smoke, 16
circulation, poor, 189
cold intolerance, 78
cold sores, 148
colitis, 25
collagen, 23, 28, 65, 146
concentrate, inability to, 188
copper, 17
cystathione synthase, 74
cysteine, 15, 23, 26, 27, 32, 133, 142, 143, 145, 146, 147, 154, 156
cystic fibrosis, 27
cystine, 26